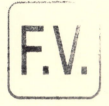

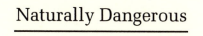

Naturally Dangerous

Naturally Dangerous

SURPRISING FACTS ABOUT FOOD,
HEALTH, AND THE ENVIRONMENT

James P. Collman

PROFESSOR OF CHEMISTRY
DEPARTMENT OF CHEMISTRY
STANFORD UNIVERSITY

University Science Books
Sausalito, California

University Science Books
55D Gate Five Road
Sausalito, CA 94965
www.uscibooks.com
Order Information:
    Phone (703) 661- 1572
    Fax (703) 661-1501

Cover cartoon reproduced with permission from the copyright
holder, Sidney Harris.

Production Manager: *Susanna Tadlock*
Designer: *Robert Ishi*
Compositor: *BookMatters*
Printer and Binder: *Maple-Vail Book Manufacturing Group*

This book is printed on acid-free paper.

Library of Congress Cataloging-in-Publication Data

Collman, James Paddock, 1932-
        Naturally dangerous : surprising facts about food,
health, and the environment / James P. Collman.
            p. cm.
        Includes bibliographical references and index.
        ISBN 1-891389-09-2
        1. Food contamination. 2. Food additives. I. Title.

        TX531.C58 2000
        363.19'26—dc21   00-049743

Printed in the United States of America
10 9 8 7 6 5 4 3 2

Contents

Contents

Preface

This book has been written so that it can be understood by all readers—nonscientists, engineers, physicians, and scientists alike. Other than a few molecular formulas such as H_2O and O_2, there are no long chemical formulas, nor is there any math. The material included should be of interest to everyone because it relates to molecules and phenomena that affect our everyday lives. You will find surprising things: little-known facts about organic and commercial foods, natural herbs, modern medicine, and the environment. Interesting historical facts behind certain issues are sprinkled in the text. For example, did you know that George Washington gained advantage over the British forces by inoculating his troops with live smallpox virus? You will also discover that nothing is completely safe nor risk-free, even natural substances. For example, ingestion of grapefruit juice may be much more hazardous for certain people than ingestion of pesticide residues. You will encounter the recurring theme that, in many situations involving real or purported health risks, there is no "free lunch," or perfect solution, but that choices must be made balancing one risk against another.

This account includes many fascinating subjects, perhaps too many to digest by reading the book from beginning to end. The good news is that you can start anywhere and move about the book, as the chapters each stand alone. The Contents and Index both should help guide you in browsing or reviewing topics that interest you. Scientific terms are defined in the Glossary. For those who want more information or original sources, a Further Reading list is included at the end, organized by chapter. After reading this book, I hope you will recommend it to your friends and neighbors.

— *J. Collman*

Acknowledgments

I am indebted to the following people who read sections of this book or its earlier, unpublished version and offered helpful suggestions. This group includes scientists, engineers, physicians, and nonscientists: Carl Barrelet, Dorothy Baumgarten, the late Chet Berry, Dick Blois, Kate Brauman, Roman Boulatov, Art Charette, Carolyn Collman, Vicki Collman, Sandy Dornbusch, Lei Fu, Paul Herrmann, Bill Kays, William F. Little, the late Harry Mosher, John Reinan, David Riggs, Doug Skoog, Orland Soave, Kira Weissman, and Dick Zare. I also want to thank Ann McGuire, Jane Ellis, Bruce Armbruster, and other members of University Science Books for their efforts in transforming a crude manuscript into a finished book.

Illustration Credits

Naturally Dangerous

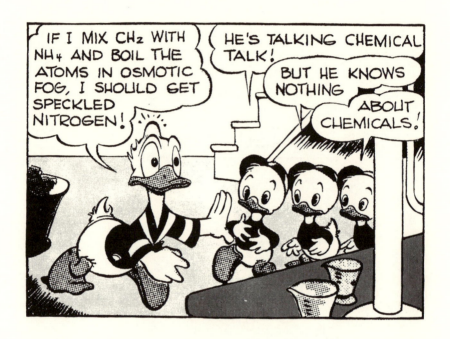

Scientific illiteracy is everywhere!

OVERTURE

Is Anything Safe?

MANY AMERICANS are under the mistaken impression that if something is "natural," it is safe. Perhaps this is the reason many people like the idea of organic foods; they are afraid of synthetic insect repellents or herbicides in commercial foods. Because of possible bacterial contamination, however, some organic foods are not entirely safe. Many substances found in nature can be deadly. Eating wild mushrooms, for example, can be fatal.

I have written this little book for intelligent, curious nonscientists to provide them with sobering facts about food, health, and the environment. If you think that organic foods or herbal medicines are completely safe, or if you believe in nuclear-free zones, read on. You will learn that some organic foods are potentially more hazardous than foods treated with pesticides. You may be surprised to discover that even everyday munchies such as potato chips and french fries contain hazardous, unnatural, *trans* fats.

To some degree, almost everything has the potential to be toxic, even those substances we require for life, such as oxygen. In this book, you will also discover that all humans are radioactive and that we emit thousands of high-energy gamma rays per minute. Perhaps you are curious about the science and the hype behind global warming and the ozone hole. Is the sky truly falling? You will discover that most of these issues are complex and there is no simple solution or "free lunch." Let's begin with toxic chemicals. The story goes back many years.

Since the days of Paracelsus, a German physician–scientist of the 16th century, doctors and chemists have known that the effect of a substance on the human body, be it good or ill, depends on the concentration in which it is taken. In the latter part of the 20th century, this bit of common sense gave way to an irrational fear of "chemicals," in particular, of anything that is not natural. Fear of cancer and of carcinogenic (cancer-causing) substances has become especially acute.

In the following accounts, you will see that these fears are not always based on sound scientific principles and are causing economic and even medical harm. At present, many people are ingesting large amounts of unstudied, natural herbal medicines, some of which can be dangerous. Don't be fooled by the word *natural*. Natural is not synonymous with *safe*. Arsenic, pennyroyal, botulism toxin, and urushiol (the rash-inducing substance in poison ivy) are all natural—and are highly poisonous.

The general public is frequently assailed by news reports concerning dangerous, toxic chemicals. The public is also led to believe that only natural substances are safe and that synthetic additives and agrochemical residues are dangerous. Such reports rarely present balanced analyses of the science underlying these complex issues.

This book attempts to probe some of these issues and to put them in a more balanced perspective. The underlying origins and degree of hazards are analyzed. Two themes emerge from this analysis: (a) nothing is absolutely safe; both natural and artificial chemicals can be dangerous; and (b) the safety and/or effectiveness of any particular substance varies with its concentration and with which part of the body is exposed. For example, an additive in many ice creams could give you emphysema if it reached your lungs, but it is safe to ingest.

You may know that cyanide is poisonous. The toxicity of cyanide is well understood. This chemical blocks the major enzyme, cytochrome oxidase, that all aerobic organisms require for respiration. But did you know that cyanide occurs naturally in certain foods and in herbal remedies that can be purchased in grocery and health-food stores? Cyanide from these natural sources is not necessarily toxic. It is the *concentration* that makes cyanide lethal.

Exaggerated Health Scares and Scientific Ignorance

To illustrate how scientific illiteracy affects public opinion on what is hazardous, consider the following story reported on the Urban Legends website (www.snopes2.com). A high-school student distributed a warning about a widely used chemical, "dihydrogen monoxide," a colorless and tasteless substance that causes thousands of deaths annually. The warning noted that the compound also causes severe hydration and frequent urination, can cause sweating and vomiting, and in its gaseous state, can cause severe burns. Included was the statement, "Accidental inhalation can kill you!" and the facts that the substance has been found in tumors of terminal cancer patients, contributes to soil erosion, and is a major component of acid rain. (The student did not mention that this chemical is present in the bodies of all living people, sick or not, nor that the most common way it can kill people is by drowning.)

When 50 recipients of the notice were asked if they would support a ban of this chemical, 43 said yes, 6 were undecided, and only 1 knew that the chemical was water!

Jane Brody, a highly respected science writer for *The New York Times,* reported the following unfounded or overblown health scares. Alar, a chemical used to synchronize the ripening of apples, was denounced in 1989 on the television program *60 Minutes.* An environmental activist group supported by the actress Meryl Streep claimed alar was "the most potent cancer-causing agent in our food supply" and was a cause of childhood cancer. Immediately, alarmed parents dumped huge quantities of apples and apple juice and cost the apple industry about $375 million in lost purchases. As a result of this panic, alar was removed from the market by its manufacturer. Subsequent tests by the National Cancer Institute and the Environmental Protection Agency failed to show alar caused cancer except in doses between 100,000 and 200,000 times the normal amount a child might consume in a day's ration of apple products. In this book, you will discover that unpasteurized apple juice can be dangerous to children and adults—because of bacterial contamination from cow manure!

Overture

In 1981, an article in the *New England Journal of Medicine* by Harvard University researchers reported a connection between coffee consumption and pancreatic cancer, a universally fatal disease. This conclusion was based on a flawed study. Five years later, the same group repeated its study and failed to find evidence for such a linkage. Coffee drinkers and Starbucks relaxed.

In 1990, a study seemed to indicate an increased incidence of cancer in children whose mothers had used electric blankets, a source of electromagnetic fields (EMFs), during pregnancy. This study seemed to confirm a 1979 report hinting at a possible relationship between childhood cancer and living near high-current power lines, which emit EMFs. As a result, a warning label was placed on electric blankets, and these products were redesigned to reduce their emission of EMFs. A 1996 report issued by the National Academy of Sciences concluded that, although EMFs appear capable of affecting biological tissues, their link to cancer is unproven.

Cellular phones also produce EMFs. Claims that cellular phone use contributed to brain tumors prompted manufacturers to sponsor independent safety studies, which have not yet linked cellular phones to cancer. The greatest hazard is accidents caused by drivers using cell phones while driving.

Asbestos removal has become a major health scare, costing billions of dollars. Before 1973, asbestos was used as an insulator against fire in many public schools. Later, the Environmental Protection Agency banned the use of asbestos in schools to reduce children's exposure to this cancer-causing agent. Congressional bills in the 1980s required schools to inspect for asbestos and to remove it. Many experts believe that, although asbestos presents a minimal threat while left in place, its removal, which results in increased airborne asbestos particles, creates a much greater hazard—at a cost of more than $6 billion!

The media constantly report claims of toxic substances in foods and beverages. Which of these claims are true? The following chapters should give you a better perspective on these issues.

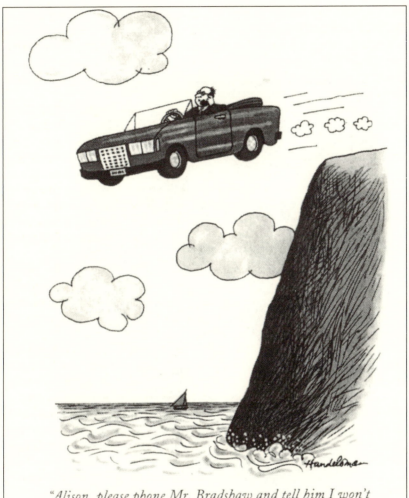

"*Alison, please phone Mr. Bradshaw and tell him I won't be available for lunch. Then call the Coast Guard and tell them I'm drowning near Long Branch, New Jersey.*"

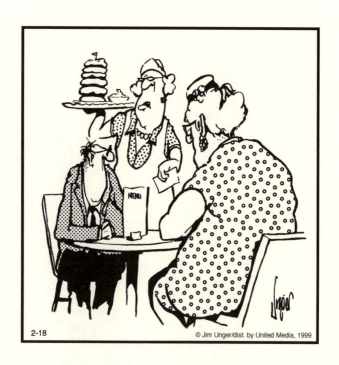

"Who gets the triple 'jumbo burger'?

1

Chemicals Lurking in Your Grocery Store

T HE FOOD WE EAT is composed of both natural and artificial chemicals. All foods are made up of chemical molecules that we put into our bodies every day. Most food molecules have a specific spatial orientation, or "handedness." Our bodies can digest only molecules that have natural handed shapes. This is the reason you should eat natural food. You may be surprised to learn that many synthetic molecules are present in a wide variety of packaged foods. Your body is not equipped to digest or metabolize these artificial foods. Many individuals who are concerned with eating only "natural foods" may be unaware of the unnatural, and possibly harmful, chemicals they unknowingly consume each day, such as those in "partially hydrogenated vegetable oils." More information about the possible dangers of these and many other food chemicals follows below. But first you should learn some basics about the major food types.

Proteins and Amino Acids

Proteins represent one of the three important classes of food molecules. Proteins are giant molecules (polymers) made by linking together large numbers of amino acids. All proteins are made up of the same natural amino acids. We need to consume these amino acid building blocks so we can produce our own proteins. Our muscles, organs, blood cells, skin, hair, and even our teeth and bones are largely made of proteins.

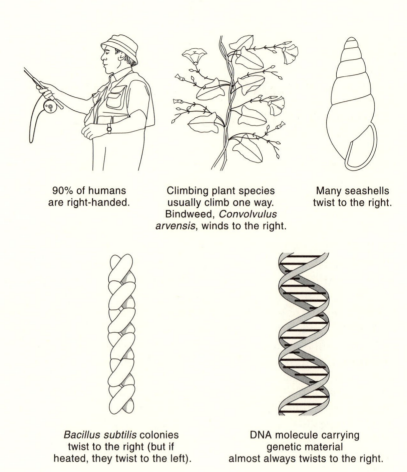

90% of humans
are right-handed.

Climbing plant species
usually climb one way.
Bindweed, *Convolvulus
arvensis*, winds to the right.

Many seashells
twist to the right.

Bacillus subtilis colonies
twist to the right (but if
heated, they twist to the left).

DNA molecule carrying
genetic material
almost always twists to the right.

Figure 1. Handedness exists in small molecules, large biomolecules such as DNA and proteins, and many living organisms, including humans. Their mirror images are not superimposable.

Throughout nature, in bacteria, plants, and animals alike, 20 different amino acids are used to make proteins. Of the 20 natural amino acids, 19 are "left handed," whereas the remaining amino acid, glycine, is not handed at all. It is amazing that all of the amino acids found in nature have the same handedness (Figure 1). Scientists call this phenomenon *homochirality.* The shapes and biological activities of proteins depend on the uniform left-handed structures of the amino acid building blocks. You cannot digest proteins made from right-handed amino acids because your enzymes will not accept these unnatural molecules. Scientists are uncertain about the origin of homochirality. One explanation is that homochirality originally came to Earth from outer space! Evidence in support of this hypothesis was found by examining amino acids extracted from a meteorite that fell near Murchison, Australia, in 1969. An elevated ratio of left-handed to right-handed amino acids was found in the carbon-rich Murchison meteorite. Isotopic analysis demonstrated that these amino acids came from outer space.

Plants make amino acids and proteins using the essential nutrient ammonia, which the plant takes up from the soil. Animals, including humans, break down, or digest, plant proteins and convert them into individual amino acids; these amino acids are then transformed into the proteins that the animal requires. Animals also manufacture some of their amino acids by breaking down and reassembling proteins in their diet. But this system is imperfect.

Essential amino acids

Bacteria can synthesize the entire set of 20 amino acids, but higher animals cannot. For example, adult humans manufacture only 12 of these 20 natural amino acids within their bodies. The other 8, called essential amino acids, must be obtained from proteins in your diet. The 20 essential and nonessential natural amino acids are listed in Table 1. One important essential amino acid, lysine, is found in corn but not in sorghum. A lysine supplement derived from corn is added to cattle, pig, and chicken feed because these animals, like humans, also lack the biochemical machinery to synthesize lysine. For this reason, corn is an important food grain for animals (and vegetarians), but as you will see, corn alone is not sufficient.

A dietary deficiency of the essential amino acid tryptophan can lead to *pellagra,* a condition characterized by dermatitis (pellagra means "rough skin"), diarrhea, and dementia. Tryptophan is converted in the body to the vitamin *niacin.* The mental difficulties in dementia probably result from a deficiency of essential brain chemicals such as the "feel good" molecule, serotonin, that the body makes from tryptophan. Corn is deficient in tryptophan and contains little useful niacin. In the 1800s, populations in Egypt and other parts of

Table 1   Essential and nonessential amino acids

Nonessential	Essential
Alanine	Isoleucine
Arginine	Leucine
Asparagine	Lysine
Aspartate	Methionine
Cysteine	Phenylalanine
Glutamate	Threonine
Glutamine	Tryptophan
Glycine	Valine
Histidine*	
Proline	
Serine	
Tyrosine	

*Essential for infants only.

Africa suffered epidemics of pellagra. In the 1930s depression, 200,000 sharecroppers in the southern United States experienced this dietary disease.

Too much of certain amino acids can be deleterious. For instance, an excess of tryptophan is not good for people who suffer from migraines; tryptophan-rich foods such as nuts are thought to trigger migraine headaches in susceptible individuals. A high level of a modified amino acid made in the body, homocysteine, is an indicator of possible heart problems.

Typical dietary sources of protein are meat, fish, milk, eggs, legumes, and cereal grains (including rice). All animal foods—meat, eggs, and milk products—are complete protein sources (i.e., they contain all the essential amino acids). This is because all animals have the same biochemical requirements. Plant sources are usually incomplete protein sources because some essential amino acids are often missing. Soybean products (e.g., tofu) are nearly complete, but, as mentioned above, corn protein is incomplete so that corn products alone cannot sustain life. Whole grains, beans, and nuts are barely adequate as protein sources; vegetarians and especially pregnant women need to be aware of this problem. By eating complementary

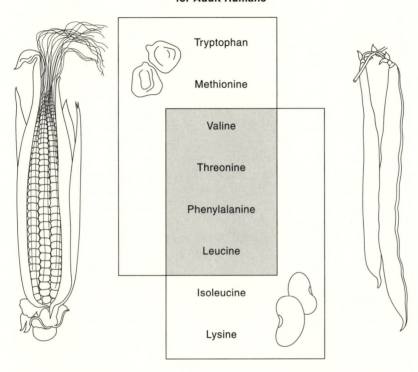

The Eight Essential Amino Acids for Adult Humans

Tryptophan

Methionine

Valine

Threonine

Phenylalanine

Leucine

Isoleucine

Lysine

Corn and other grains

Beans and other legumes

Figure 2. The availability of essential amino acids in a vegetable diet. Tryptophan and methionine are abundant in corn but are missing in beans. In contrast, corn has little isoleucine and lysine, while beans are rich in these nutrients. All eight essential amino acids can be obtained by consuming a meal of corn and beans.

plant proteins in tandem, you can obtain a complete stock of the essential amino acids. Thus, corn plus pinto beans (an American Indian staple), or rice and soybeans (a traditional Asian diet), or peas or lentils together with wheat or barley (a combination eaten in prehistoric Europe) afford the proper balance of essential amino acids. Figure 2 illustrates an example of such balanced use of vegetables.

Protein diets

The recommended daily protein intake for adult men is about 60 grams (2.1 oz.); for women, it is 50 grams, unless they are pregnant or breastfeeding, in which case 60 to 65 grams are recommended. The amount of required protein depends to a certain extent on body weight. People in developing nations get by with less protein, consuming approximately 40 grams per person. Too much protein intake carries potential risks, such as kidney damage.

A high-protein, high-fat, low-carbohydrate diet has been in vogue recently in developed countries; in fact, this scheme was first promulgated in 1863 by a British undertaker, William Banting. This low-carbohydrate diet is a gimmick that apparently is not supported by any careful scientific study. Weight loss does occur with limited carbohydrate intake, but it is largely the result of a loss of water because carbohydrates are the nutrients that hold water in your body. One gram of water is stored with every gram of carbohydrate. Substances called ketones accumulate in the bloodstream when the body is low in carbohydrates. This accumulation can make a person light-headed and nauseated, and it can cause bad breath. This diet can also lead to potassium, sodium, and calcium loss, which raises the risk of osteoporosis. Another side effect is an increase in uric acid, a phenomenon that can cause kidney stones to develop.

The dietary requirements of animals are often different from those of humans. A couple of examples may be of interest. Certain animals subsist on a high-protein diet from ingesting food such as insects. Trout, for example, feed almost entirely on insect life. Also, a black bear's diet throughout the year consists of 10% insects from sources such as ants, termites, and yellow jackets.

Carbohydrates

Almost everyone has heard the terms sugars and carbohydrates, but people do not realize that these are related. All carbohydrates are made up of sugar units the way proteins are made up of amino acid units. In fact, many food labels separate sugar and carbohydrate contents in food products. Carbohydrates are one of the major classes of biomolecules, along with proteins, discussed above, and fats, described below.

Simple carbohydrates are made of one or two rings of carbon attached to oxygen and hydrogen; they are often referred to as sugars. Giant polymers of these sugars are called complex carbohydrates. Starch and cellulose (from plants) are examples of polymeric sugars. We are able to digest starch but not cellulose.

Sugar molecules are covered with multiple hydroxyl, or OH groups, making them soluble in water but insoluble in oil. The best known and most important sugar is glucose, whose molecular formula can be written as $[C(H_2O)]_n$. The term *carbohydrate* (hydrate of carbon) derives from the molecular composition of carbohydrates.

Carbohydrates have multiple roles in all forms of life; consequently, they make up most of the organic matter on Earth. Carbohydrates serve as energy stores, fuels, and metabolic intermediates. Starch in plants, and a similar substance, glycogen, in animals, can be rapidly converted into glucose, which is the primary fuel used to generate energy in our bodies. Glycogen, a chain of glucose molecules (a polysaccharide), is stored in the muscle cells of animals. When we exercise, we consume our supplies of glucose and glycogen, but little fat is metabolized.

Many other sugar derivatives are essential components of living systems. For example, the sugars ribose and deoxyribose form the structural framework of the genetic molecules RNA and DNA, respectively. Polysaccharides such as cellulose are the structural elements of cell walls in plants and bacteria, as well as in the shells of arthropods such as crabs and lobsters.

The most common sugar in our diet, sucrose, is somewhat complicated. Sucrose consists of two simple sugars, glucose and fructose, linked together. Such sugars are called disaccharides (literally, two sugars). One well-known disaccharide is lactose, which is found in milk.

Sucrose is obtained commercially from sugar cane (Figure 3, see color section), which grows only in the tropics, or from sugar beets, which will grow in more moderate climates such as that of eastern Colorado. Cane sugar was imported into Europe from India after Roman times (the Romans relied on honey as a sweetener). Napoleon promoted the production of beet sugar to get around the British blockade. Economically, sucrose from beets cannot compete with sugar from cane, but beet sugar is subsidized by price supplements and price controls, and is thus a classic "political commodity." Without these controls or import duties, it is doubtful that sugar beets would be grown commercially in the United States, and you would pay much less for sugar. Because of various price controls, you pay an artificially high price for sugar and all products made from sugar. The public is not widely aware of this fact.

Fructose is obtained commercially by the use of enzymes acting on corn starch. Fructose is 1.75 times sweeter per unit weight than sucrose is. This fructose-rich corn syrup is added to many soft drinks (I personally find it too sweet). Fructose is the principal sugar in honey.

Lactose is the disaccharide present in milk, both human and bovine. It is composed of two different monosaccharides, glucose and galactose. To be digested, milk sugar must be broken down into these two monosaccharide components. Nearly all infants and children are able to digest milk sugar; however, many adults in the world experience stomach cramps and diarrhea after they ingest lactose from consuming too much milk and other dairy products such as ice cream.

Why is this true, when so many readers of this book probably eat ice cream without experiencing any digestive upset? The answer depends on your genetic makeup. The digestive splitting of lactose is catalyzed by an enzyme called lactase. Many individuals lose their ability to digest dairy products as they enter adulthood, because their body no longer produces lactase. Lactase-deficient people are said to be lactose intolerant. Interestingly, most people from central and northern Europe continue to make the enzyme lactase as they enter adulthood and therefore can drink milk comfortably throughout their lifetimes. These people are descendants of a population that domesticated cattle some 10,000 years ago, just after the last ice age. The genetic difference may be related to the amount of sunlight various populations are exposed to; peoples in regions of the Earth with lower amounts of sunlight may have relied on milk products for some of their vitamin D and therefore needed lactase in adulthood. Human populations that historically did not consume milk in adulthood generally have a higher incidence of lactase deficiency. For example, 97% of Thais are deficient in lactase compared with only 3% of Danes. Incidentally, there is little lactose in cheese or yogurt, so lactase-deficient people can digest these milk products.

Some lactose-intolerant adults add lactase to their milk or more commonly buy lactose-free dairy products. If you taste such milk, you will find it to be sweet, because the two monosaccharides resulting from the breakdown of lactose are sweeter than the disaccharide. For some, there is an interesting lesson here. Lactase-treated milk is an unnatural mixture of natural sugars, and it is a healthful food; whereas lactose, a natural sugar, is unhealthful for many individuals. This example shows that "natural" is not always the safest.

Artificial sweeteners

Artificial sweeteners are synthetic chemicals, not sugars at all. They are unnatural molecules that cause a sweet sensation but are not metabolized, and thus add no calories to our bodies. Their most important use is by diabetics, who must control their intake of sucrose, fructose, and glucose. However, their major use is by people looking to cut their intake of calories. There is big money to be made in the sale of artificial sweeteners, but the costs associated with obtaining approval from the US Food and Drug Administration are considerable. This large, long-term investment must be followed by manufacture and marketing, which are also very expensive.

The oldest accepted synthetic sweetener is saccharin, which is 300 times as sweet as table sugar. Saccharin's bitter aftertaste makes it a less desirable product, however. Even though saccharin had been produced commercially since 1900, its use was later challenged because it was found to be a mild carcinogen, and in relatively high concentrations have been reported to cause cancer in the bladders of rats. Promoters of saccharin argued that the research was not directly applicable to humans because rats concentrate their urine more than humans do. The proponents of saccharin won, and the substance is still permitted to be sold as an artificial sweetener. In 2000, the US government removed saccharin from its list of carcinogens. It is interesting that honey bees will not eat saccharin; neither will your author.

Cyclamate was once widely used as a sweetener in the United States in soft drinks, canned fruits, candy, and salad dressings. Cyclamate is 30 times as sweet as table sugar, and it tastes better than saccharin to most people, including your author. By 1969, 21 million pounds of cyclamate were sold annually in the United States, but in 1970, it was banned as a suspected carcinogen. This finding was, unfortunately, the result of bad science. The actual cancer-causing agent in the animal tests was later discovered to be an impurity that is not present in commercial samples of cyclamate. Despite this finding, cyclamate has not been permitted back on the US market, even though it is used in several foreign countries, including Canada. A request for reapproval filed in 1985 is still pending.

Presently, the most popular and widely used artificial sweetener in the United States is marketed as NutraSweet and Equal. This synthetic chemical contains an active ingredient called aspartame, a proteinlike molecule formed from two naturally occurring amino acids, aspartic acid and phenylalanine. Many of the young people I've known consume NutraSweet in diet soft drinks. This substance is 100 to 200 times sweeter than table sugar and does not have a bitter aftertaste like saccharin. Aspartame has an Achilles' heel in that it contains an amide link, like all proteins, and such bonds are not stable in water. Although the rate of aspartame's breakdown into its separate amino acids is slow under mild conditions, in hot, acidic solutions, the rate is much more rapid. If the breakdown of amide bonds in proteins were normally this rapid, our hands, which are largely protein, would dissolve when we washed them. Because the active ingredient in aspartame decomposes in water, diet drinks containing NutraSweet (or Equal) have a limited shelf life—especially if they are stored at high temperatures without refrigeration. Remember that a manufacturer has no control over what customers do with their diet-drink cans, nor do consumers know the storage history of the drinks they buy. A somewhat more serious problem is that aspartame cannot withstand some cooking or baking conditions without breaking down, which makes the sweetness disappear because the resulting amino acids are bitter. Cakes and other sweet baked goods therefore cannot be made using this artificial sweetener.

One of the by-products from digesting NutraSweet or Equal is the natural amino acid phenylalanine. Critics believe that the consumption of NutraSweet or Equal can be dangerous to the few people, roughly 1 in 15,000, who have a metabolic disorder known as phenylketonuria, or PKU. These individuals lack an enzyme needed to process the phenylalanine, and concentrations can reach toxic levels in their blood and cause mental retardation unless dietary sources of this amino acid are restricted. Each package of NutraSweet and Equal contains a warning label to this effect. Many people who avoid chemicals and favor natural foods may not realize that diet drinks contain a synthetic chemical that is possibly hazardous.

Bread and Cereals

Baked goods and cereals made from grain are considered among the most healthful foods, but this is not true for everyone. Some individuals have an inherited disorder called Celiac Sprue, which is the result of an abnormal immune response to ingestion of proteins, like gluten, that are found in wheat, rye, oats, barley, and other similar grains, but not in rice. This disorder affects about 1 in 25,000 people, principally those of European ancestry; approximately 70% of the cases occur in women. Celiac Sprue is rather common in Wales, where 1 in 600 are said to be affected.

Symptoms of Celiac Sprue include weight loss, anemia, vitamin deficiencies, weakness, fatigue, finger numbness, and inability to concentrate. This disorder can be fatal, especially to infants. The diagnosis is often missed in the United States, where physicians are less aware of it. Once diagnosed, Celiac Sprue can be controlled simply by a life-long, gluten-free diet. Soy and rice products can be substituted for the traditional Western grains. Those with the disease may drink rice beer rather than that made from grain.

Fats

Every day we hear about fat in our diet. One must worry about saturated versus unsaturated fat, as well as new synthetic fats (fat substitutes). But what *is* fat, and how do our bodies use it? Fats belong to a larger class of biomolecules, called lipids. Lipids are water-insoluble biomolecules that are soluble in organic solvents such as chloroform. In living systems, lipids serve as energy-storage compounds, as fuel molecules, and as the major components of biological membranes, including the delicate membranes surrounding all cells.

The most important building blocks of lipids are the fatty acids. The 16- and 18-carbon fatty acids are the most common; the hydrocarbon chain may be saturated (i.e., contains no carbon–carbon double bonds) or it may be unsaturated (i.e., contains one or more dou-

healthful. There is one naturally occurring *trans* fatty acid in food. Buttermilk and other animal fats contain small amounts of vaccenic acid, a natural *trans* fatty acid. The consequences of consuming vaccenic acid are presently unknown.

Some medical scientists believe that the *trans* double bonds in chemically modified fats are potentially dangerous; your enzymes are not designed to metabolize molecules that have *trans* double bonds! An ample body of evidence now implicates *trans* fats in heart disease. *Trans* fats appear to interfere with the metabolism of polyunsaturated fatty acids, which are thought to protect against arterial clogging and heart disease. Other epidemiologic evidence implicates *trans* fats in a higher incidence of breast cancer. A European study of about 700 postmenopausal women found those whose bodies contained the highest levels of *trans* fatty acids were 40% more likely to develop breast cancer than were women who had the lowest levels.

To avoid eating *trans* fatty acids, which also elevate cholesterol levels, you should avoid eating products marked as containing partially hydrogenated fat or high levels of hydrogenated vegetable oil. This ingredient is difficult to avoid because hard margarine, Crisco, cakes, pies, candy bars, crackers, cookies, and several types of potato chips contain this unnatural food. This potential problem received scant attention in the media until 2000, when the government proposed labeling food products containing *trans* fats. Could that omission be explained by the huge commercial resources that have an interest in selling hydrogenated vegetable oils?

Here's a kicker: the consumption of certain margarines actually cuts your cholesterol level! These margarines are not made from partially hydrogenated vegetable oils, but instead they contain sterols, natural chemicals derived from soybeans. Sterols are thought to "masquerade" as cholesterol in the body and interfere with cholesterol absorption. These products are not yet approved for general use, but related margarines containing similar chemicals, stanols, derived from wood pulp of pine trees have been used for many years in Finland and are now approved for sale in the United States. Use of these stanol-containing margarines is claimed to lower the level of LDL, the bad cholesterol. However, about 70% of the margarine sold in the United States is made from partially hydrogenated vegetable oil and contains potentially hazardous *trans* fats.

Chemicals Lurking in Your Grocery

Fat substitutes

In 1996, the FDA approved a fat substitute, called olestra, for use in salty snacks such as potato chips, tortilla chips, and crackers. Olestra, sold under the brand name Olean, is the result of a $200 to $300 million testing program by Proctor and Gamble. The major component, olestin, is a derivative of table sugar, sucrose, combined with fatty acid esters. This artificial chemical travels through the body without being adsorbed or digested, thus leaving no calories behind. The enzymes in your body are not able to interact with this unnatural substance, but it gives your mouth the feel of a fat. The justification for adding olestra to food products stems from the large amount of natural fatty foods many Americans consume. Proctor and Gamble estimates that Americans eat 5.5 billion pounds of snack food each year—22 pounds per person on average. Many of these snack foods are prepared by cooking in fat, which in many instances is partially hydrogenated fat. One out of three Americans is obese.

Fat substitutes like olestra may not be risk-free; they dissolve and therefore deplete the body of the fat-soluble vitamins A, D, E, and K. Because of this concern, the FDA has required that olestra-containing foods be fortified with those vitamins. There might still be a risk for "bleeders," people who are very sensitive to fluctuations in vitamin K (which is associated with blood clotting) such as those taking "blood-thinning" medicines such as heparin and coumadin. Other critics of olestra are concerned with its potential depletion of carotenoids, which are thought to help ward off heart disease, strokes, and possibly cancer. Olestra will apparently not be fortified with carotenoids. Other annoying side effects of olestra are nausea, stomach cramps, and diarrhea ("anal drip"). These effects may limit public acceptance of this food additive that has negative nutritional value.

Additional fat substitutes that are derived from foodstuffs are appearing on the market. For example, Oatrim and Nu-Trim are products made from oats. These substances are claimed to reduce cholesterol levels in hamsters and might therefore be healthful in people. Nu-Trim is said to mimic the texture and mouth feel of fat without the calories of natural fats.

Chocolate

Do you crave chocolate? Chocolate is said to be truly addictive to a small percentage of the population—more often women. Why might chocolate be addictive? To answer this question, you need to know a little more about chocolate. Neither the sugar nor the milk added to milk chocolate is thought to be the hedonistic agent responsible for chocolate's rare, addictive character. One addictive ingredient in chocolate, however, the alkaloid theobromine (a nitrogen-containing ring compound), has a chemical structure very similar to that of caffeine—the stimulant found in coffee and teas. This and some other chemicals in chocolate bind to the same brain receptor systems targeted by marijuana!

Chocolate was a gift from the New World to the Old; it is derived from the seeds (cocoa beans) of the tree *Theobroma cacao* (Figure 4, see color section). This name derives from the Greek word for "food of the Gods." Although this plant is indigenous to the Amazon, 65% of the world's cacao is now produced in west Africa. Christopher Columbus found that the Aztecs drank a bitter preparation from the cacao bean. The Aztecs held this drink in high regard despite its bitter taste. Aztec nobles regarded chocolate as an aphrodisiac. Columbus introduced chocolate to Europe in 1502, but chocolate became popular in Europe only after the Spanish learned to sweeten it. By 1751, London had 2,000 chocolate houses.

Chocolate is prepared by fermenting the cacao bean. This enzyme-catalyzed process hydrolyzes and oxidizes proteins in the bean, thus developing chocolate's distinctive flavor. This process possibly releases exorphins, which are peptides (small protein fragments) that act like endorphins. The latter are pleasure-giving peptides naturally produced in the brain. Enzymatic cleavage of proteins including those found in milk, gluten (a protein in wheat), certain meat products, and several other foodstuffs can also produce exorphins. The small exorphin peptides (four or five amino-acid units) bind to the same receptors in the brain that morphine and other opium components do. The action of exorphins is blocked by a molecule, naloxone, that is an opiate antagonist (antidote). It has been suggested that exorphins produced from the enzymatic digestion of milk in the stomach may provide a reward to an infant, rein-forcing the desire to nurse, increasing mother–child bonding, and in-ducing sleep. Are such exorphins also responsible for the chocolate "highs" experienced by a few susceptible individuals with the cor-rect enzymes? The answer remains uncertain.

Chocolate is widely believed to trigger migraine headaches. Not to worry! In 1998, a study of 63 women plagued with chronic head-aches pretty much exonerated chocolate from the charge of inducing headaches, even migraines. A common belief is that women crave chocolate more than men do. Although this may be true for Americans, Spanish women do not have any more interest in choco-late than Spanish men do. This difference suggests that the prefer-ence is cultural rather than gender-based.

There is other good news for chocolate lovers. Chocolate contains hefty quantities of natural antioxidants called flavonoids. These com-pounds, also found in tea and red wine, are associated with a reduced risk of cardiovascular disease. A small cup of milk chocolate typically contains about the same quantity of antioxidant as a glass of red wine. A serving of dark chocolate contains twice that amount—roughly the same quantity as a cup of black tea. There are several types of flavo-noids in chocolate. Some of these exert other effects, in addition to the antioxidant roles. For example, certain flavonoids help relax the inner surface of blood vessels by increasing concentrations of nitric oxide, an important hormone. Chocolate appears to be another nutriceutical, a food offering health benefits. To some it is far more palatable than broccoli.

Asparagus

Does your urine have an odor just after you eat asparagus? If so, you are not alone, but not everyone experiences this result. The odor is caused by sulfur-containing metabolites, or breakdown products, produced in the body from constituents in the asparagus. This phe-nomenon was not noted before the late 17th century, when sulfur and sulfur compounds were added as fertilizer to improve asparagus flavor. The ability to carry out the required metabolism to produce the odor is inherited, a dominant genetic trait with no apparent gender distinction. Many men believed this odor production to be a male trait—not so. There seems, however, to be national variation. For example, only about 40% of the 915 test subjects in the United Kingdom produced the odor, whereas in another study, all 103 French citizens did. In contrast, only 10% of 307 volunteer "sniffers" were able to detect high dilutions of urine from asparagus-eating donors. Seemingly, the heightened sense of smell and the enzymatic production of the smell are not genetically correlated. This natural odor is not considered toxic.

Foods Rich in Oxalate

Every year, some 500,000 Americans experience painful kidney stones; about 70% are men. Those at highest risk of a future attack have already endured the excruciating pain from a kidney stone, and must control their diets. The principal mineral in kidney stones is calcium, combined with oxalate. People who have experienced a calcium oxalate kidney stone have an intrinsic, possibly inherited, metabolic problem and should avoid foods that are rich in oxalate; rhubarb, spinach, beets, sweet potatoes, parsley, nuts, instant coffee, tea, and chocolate are on the list (Table 2). Surprisingly, even though a high level of calcium in the urine is a predictor of kidney stones, people who have had such stones are encouraged to eat moderate amounts of foods rich in calcium (e.g., milk, cheese, yogurt, oranges, and broccoli). These dietary calcium foods do not cause kidney stones. Calcium and vitamin D supplements, however, should be avoided by susceptible individuals. This example is an excellent illustration of the fact that eating foods rich in a mineral is different from taking a supplement of that mineral. Another way to prevent kidney stones is simple: drink copious quantities of fluid, at least ten 8-ounce glasses per day. The fluids may be water, beer, wine, and even milk. There is an interesting point here: a subsection of the population needs to avoid common foods that are safe and nutritious to others.

Table 2   Foods for kidney stone patients to avoid

Foods of high oxalic acid content (0.1% or more)— to be avoided	Foods of moderate oxalic acid content (0.02% or more)— to be eaten sparingly
beets	beans (green and wax)
beet tops	blackberries
black tea	blueberries
chenopodium	carrots
chocolate	celery
cocoa	coffee (roasted)
dried figs	Concord grapes
ground pepper	currants (red)
lamb quarters	dandelion greens
lime peel	endive
nuts	gooseberries
parsley	lemon peel
poke	okra
poppy seeds	onions (green)
purslane	oranges
rhubarb	orange peel
sorrel	peppers (green)
spinach	strawberries
Swiss chard	sweet potatoes

Flowers

Adding flowers to food is an ancient custom. From ancient times, Chinese cooks have used chrysanthemum, lily and lotus flowers or buds in their recipes. Your garden may contain an array of edible flowers. Chrysanthemums, dandelions, daylilies, lavender, marigolds, nasturtiums, pansies, roses, scented geraniums, and sunflowers are examples of edible flowers. Some are very nutritional. Nasturtiums, for example, have high levels of vitamins A, C, and D. Edible flowers enhance salads, and they may also be used in soups, pastas, and stir fries. These attractive, natural foods can be purchased in a few select grocery stores.

Be cautious, though. Not all flowers are edible, and some are toxic! The following is an incomplete list of toxic flowers: clematis (virgin's bower), crocus, daphne, foxglove, amaryllis, cardinal flower, mistletoe, azalea (rhododendron), calla lily, and alkali grass (wild onion). Some edible flowers can cause allergies; for example, English chamomile should be avoided by people allergic to ragweed, as they may also be allergic to chamomile. If you have hayfever, asthma, or allergies, do not eat any flowers. Flowers are like wild mushrooms; some are nutritious, and others are toxic. However, only a few flowers are as deadly as poisonous mushrooms. Eat only flowers you are certain are not toxic. Personally, I eschew flowers in a homemade salad, because the preparer may not know which flowers are safe to eat, and I do not always remember which is which myself.

Vegemite

Thinly smeared on toast, this odd substance is eaten by Australians and New Zealanders. Australians consume 4,500 metric tons of vegemite annually. It is made from a yeast slurry, a brewery waste product that also does service as pig feed. The appearance of vegemite, which is similar to used chewing-tobacco, repels the uninitiated, as does its taste and smell. Australians, most of whom are introduced to vegemite in their childhood, crave its flavor, but people of other nationalities seldom taste it more than once, if that often. Neither do bacteria enjoy this natural foodstuff, as it is said not to spoil in the Outback, Australia's vast, arid interior. I know an Australian scientist who keeps a 15-year-old bottle of vegemite in his kitchen. Vegemite is an example of a natural food that is quite safe, possibly nutritious, but repugnant to most adults. I wonder if vegemite has antibiotic activity?

Spices: Ancient Herbal Antibiotics

Most of the spices or condiments we add to food are toxic—at some concentration. Before the advent of refrigeration, these natural food additives were used to keep food from decaying. Scientists now understand that these preservatives act by killing bacteria. Historically, foods were salted to inhibit decay. Some scientists now believe that excess salt could be harmful because the consumption of excess sodium ions, as in table salt, contributes to osteoporosis, stomach cancer, and kidney disease. Too much dietary salt also seems to deplete calcium levels in bones. Many physicians therefore advocate a low-salt diet.

The history of early civilizations is filled with quests for spices. Trade between the Orient and Europe was stimulated by the demand for spices. They are natural compounds that evolved in plants as protection against pathogens and predators. Spices are more prominent in dishes from tropical and subtropical regions and are used to a lesser extent, if at all, in colder climates. It has been argued that spice plants contain powerful antibiotic chemicals capable of killing or suppressing the growth of bacteria that spoil foods. Spices such as garlic, onion, and hot peppers have been found to inhibit more than 75% of the bacteria species they have been tested against. In ancient societies, spices were also used in mummification.

Spices can have a downside. Some of the antimicrobial chemicals found in spice plants, when administered in large quantities, are mutagenic (damage DNA), carcinogenic (cause cancer), or teratogenic (cause birth defects). The effects depend on the amount consumed and the circumstances. This downside may be why pregnant women and small children tend to avoid spicy foods. Most of the general public are unaware of these properties and freely use spices as natural food additives.

An interesting spice is horseradish. The active ingredient in both horseradish and mustard, allyl isothiocyanate, is an irritating substance that is dangerous if inhaled and can cause skin and eye irritation. To illustrate: a small manufacturer of LaBombard Horseradish, which comes in four varieties (Regular Hot, X Hot, XXX Hot, and Too Darn Hot) spilled 1.5 quarts of the active ingredient. After receiving an emergency phone call, firefighters turned up equipped with masks but, even so, were driven away by this pungent chemical. The same compound, allyl isothiocyanate, was once used in gas warfare! Think of that when you put horseradish on your food.

You might think that the active ingredient in chili peppers, capsaicin, might be toxic because it irritates your skin. Capsaicin affects physiological perception of pain and body temperature and has some therapeutic value in a pain-relieving ointment. Birds cannot taste capsaicin, but squirrels avoid any pepper-treated bird seeds; this trait is the basis of a patent for squirrel-proof bird seeds. There is an ultrapotent capsaicin analog that has been used as a topical pain reliever for more than 2,000 years. This compound, resiniferatoxin, or RTX, was developed in Mauritania in east Africa by King Juba II (50 B.C.–23 A.D.). In historic times, RTX was used for whimsical purposes: as a treatment for lethargy (a touch on the nostrils had dramatic results) and to provoke sneezing (until tobacco was used for this purpose). RTX has about 10,000 times the potency of capsaicin. RTX is currently being evaluated as an analgesic agent despite the fact that the resin it comes from is found only in places such as Nigeria, Iran, and Iraq.

Flavor Enhancers

Since ancient times, cooks have known that some food additives enhance or modify the taste and odor of foods. There are several such agents, but the most widely used and best known by the general public is monosodium glutamate (MSG), the sodium salt of the natural amino acid, glutamic acid. This natural substance is widely sold as a flavor enhancer and is used in many Chinese restaurants. MSG suppresses sweetness, bitterness, and the cooling effect of menthol, but it does not affect sourness or butteriness. MSG is typically used in soups, sauces, meat and fish products, and, of course, Chinese food. Many individuals believe they have a sensitivity to MSG; this sensitivity is widely referred to as "Chinese restaurant syndrome." In Australia, however, a careful, double-blind study among individuals who claimed to suffer from this syndrome did not confirm MSG as the causal agent. Perhaps other substances in Chinese food, such as allergenic proteins, food dyes, or preservatives, are responsible for the actual phenomenon. In 1991, the European Union's Scientific Committee for Food gave MSG a clean bill of health and placed this substance in the safest category for food additives.

Scientists have now uncovered one of the secrets behind the effectiveness of MSG as a flavor enhancer. Because MSG binds to a specific taste receptor for a taste called umami, it has a specific flavor. Along with the four familiar tastes—salty, sweet, sour, and bitter—umami is another basic flavor recognized by the tongue. Umami is a taste found in parmesan cheese, mushrooms, meat, and some Asian foods. In Japanese, *umami* loosely means "delicious," or "yummy."

Natural Toxins in Food
(Even Vegetables Can Be Dangerous)

There are many natural toxins in food. For example, many vegetables have developed natural insecticides to protect themselves from predators; after all, a plant cannot run away! Some of these substances are quite toxic. These natural toxic chemicals are more prevalent in foods like potatoes grown under "natural conditions" without the benefit of herbicides, because the plants respond by producing their own defenses.

The potato belongs to the nightshade family, some members of which contain naturally toxic substances. The skin of the common potato contains compounds called glycoalkaloids. Two examples are solanine and chaconine, which affect both the central nervous system and the digestive tract. For example, solanine is as poisonous as parathion, a synthetic pesticide, banned in the United States because of its high toxicity. These toxic glycoalkaloids are found in higher concentrations on potatoes that have been damaged or are bred to be disease resistant. For safety, any portion of the potato skin that is green should be removed. Generally speaking, though, potatoes are safe to eat. Unless you eat large amounts of peels from low-quality potatoes, these toxins are not a serious health hazard. Other food poisons result from fungi (molds) that occur on the plant under moist conditions. Some natural toxins are thought to be the origins of the many plagues that were reported in earlier times, including some referred to in the Bible.

Chemicals Lurking in Your Grocery Store

Another natural toxin that is unknown to the general public is found in umbellaferae plants, such as celery and parsnips. During World War I, soldiers unloading supplies of these herbs came down with painful skin inflammations. Gardeners and warehouse workers had similar problems, which arose from compounds such as one known as 5-MOP. Umbellaferae plants use these substances, collectively known as furocoumarins, as chemical weapons against microorganisms. A combination of furocoumarins and ultraviolet light was once used to treat a skin disease, but this use was found to produce cancer in animals. The World Health Organization links such treatment to skin cancer in humans.

One of the most infamous toxins that enters the food chain is aflatoxin B_1, which is produced by molds in several crops, including peanuts, corn, and even spinach. Any wet, moldy vegetable is a possible source of this dangerous substance. Scientific evidence has associated aflatoxin with an increased risk of liver cancer. The FDA limit on aflatoxin in human food is 20 parts per billion (ppb) and 100 ppb for livestock feed. Entire corn crops have been threatened by high concentrations of aflatoxin. In 1998, more than 80% of the corn crop in Texas was contaminated by this toxin. On occasion, peanut butter has been claimed to exceed the allowed limit of aflatoxin.

It has been suggested that an increased use of fungicides on food crops might reduce the risk of cancer by lowering the amount of aflatoxin produced from molds (fungi). This use of chemicals would run counter to the ideas of natural foods advocates. At the least, you should avoid moldy food; for example, I avoid eating raspberries with gray spots.

Another little-recognized natural toxin is the ethyl ester of phorbol, which is reported to be found in some herbal teas but not in traditional tea. Phorbol esters are cocarcinogens; they promote tumors and should be regarded as potentially dangerous.

As mentioned earlier, there have been many claims that coffee contains harmful substances besides the stimulant caffeine. One by one, upon further investigation, these fears have proved unfounded. Nevertheless, in 1999, a report from researchers in the Netherlands may cause some people to avoid a particular type of coffee: cafeteria or unfiltered (Turkish type) coffee. This plunger-brewed coffee retains some lipids called cafestol and kahwool, which produce increased blood levels of LDL, the "bad" cholesterol associated with an increased risk of heart disease. Filters remove these potentially harmful lipids. Cholesterol-raising effects were not found in instant coffee, which has little of these lipids, nor in Italian espresso. These researchers found that people who drink five to six cups of Turkish-type coffee per day for six months had LDL cholesterol levels raised by 9% to 14%. Choose your coffee carefully!

Some foods are actually dangerous and should not be eaten at all. For example, three commonly eaten tropical fruits—soursop, custard apple, pomme cannelle, and teas made from these fruits—may cause disorders similar to Parkinson's disease. Symptoms include incontinence, slurred speech, tremors, slowness of movement, poor balance, and loss of eyelid control. Naturally occurring neurotoxins in these plants are thought to cause these illnesses. These dangerous, natural foods cannot be purchased in American food stores, but they are sometimes available in tropical markets.

Organic Foods

Organic food, promoted by "political correctness" and some scientific misunderstandings, is a booming industry, with annual revenues in the United States of about $4.5 billion. Many customers are willing to pay higher prices for organic food grown without man-made chemical fertilizers and pesticides because they believe that such food is safer, healthier, and more friendly to the environment. People are also accustomed to associating higher prices with better quality. It is furthermore true that some organically grown fruits taste better because they are picked ripe. Many conventionally grown fruits are picked while green and are artificially ripened using a plant hormone, ethylene gas.

Several prominent food scientists have pointed out that, because of the way organic food is fertilized, with compost and manure, it is actually riskier to consume than food grown with synthetic chemicals. These natural fertilizers may infect the food with deadly bacteria that are carried in animal feces. Indeed, while there are no reports of death attributed to pesticide residues, the Centers for Disease Control (CDC) registers hundreds of deaths from foodborne diseases each year. For example, deadly new strains of foodborne bacteria such as *E. coli* O157:H7 are estimated to cause 250 deaths and 20,000 illnesses per year. Consumers of organic and natural food are 8 times as likely to be attacked by this dangerous new strain than those who eat conventionally grown foods. Organic food can also contain high levels of natural toxins (e.g., aflatoxins) and allergens. The politically correct status of organic foods may have kept the CDC and other government groups from widely discussing risks inherent in organic foods. It is perhaps fortunate that such foods constitute only a tiny fraction of the food supply.

Certain vegetables can be dangerous, especially organic vegetables. Alfalfa sprouts, a favorite salad ingredient, have caused outbreaks of illness traced to *Salmonella* and *E. coli* in their seeds, and *washing the sprouts does not help.* In healthy people, these bacteria can cause diarrhea, nausea, cramps, and fever over several days. The danger is higher for the elderly, who may have impaired immune systems. Young children also should not be fed these sprouts. Estimates are that more than 20,000 people in North America contracted salmonella infections from alfalfa sprouts in 1995. These sprouts are believed to have been the leading source of *E. coli* illness, much more than tainted ground beef, which has received wider publicity. Alfalfa sprouts have now disappeared from cafeteria food lines, but you may remember eating this natural food. In 1996, a similar problem occurred in Japan, where radish sprouts used as salad toppings are thought to have caused an outbreak of *E. coli* 0157, killing 11 people and giving diarrhea to thousands more.

Even foods not contaminated with bacteria may be hazardous. Bruce Ames, a professor at the University of California, Berkeley, developed a simple method for determining whether a chemical produces mutations in the DNA of bacteria. The Ames Test has become a universal screening technique for potential carcinogens. When this test was applied to synthetic insecticides results showed a cancer-producing potential that alarmed many people. Subsequent tests on rodents established that, at very high doses, about half these synthetic chemicals could, indeed, produce cancer. This information led the Environmental Protection Agency to limit the amount of pesticide residue allowed on food to "an acceptable level of risk"—calculated as that which causes an increase of no more than one cancer death per million people over a 70-year lifetime. The Agriculture Department examined 7,328 food items and detected excesses of synthetic insecticides and herbicides in 1.5% of these samples. The greatest "offenders" were apples, celery, and peaches. The fear generated from these reports helped stimulate the public's interest in natural foods because the latter are free of synthetic insecticides and herbicides.

Using the test for carcinogens that he invented, Ames subsequently discovered that many natural pesticides, which occur in foods, are also carcinogens! He reported that "almost every plant product in the supermarket is likely to contain natural carcinogens." When tested in high doses on animals, half of these natural plant chemicals turned out to be carcinogens. Of 64 natural plant pesticides that were tested, 35 are carcinogens! For example, more than 1,000 chemicals have been reported present in roasted coffee; 26 have been tested, and 19 of these were found to be carcinogens. Each day, an average American eats a gram and a half of such natural pesticides; this amount is more than 10,000 times higher than the residues from synthetic agricultural pesticides that he or she ingests. Forty-three foods were found to contain at least 10 parts per million of natural chemicals that have been found to be carcinogenic in high-dose rodent tests. These include many familiar foods: parsley, oregano, sage, rosemary, and thyme (notice that these are all condiments). These natural carcinogens occur at higher levels in plants that have not been protected by synthetic pesticides or herbicides. The level of natural carcinogens is especially high in plants that have been grown unprotected by herbicides over several generations. This is the reason that organic foods grown over several generations may contain larger amounts of natural carcinogens. Those plants that survive develop higher concentrations of natural pesticides. It has been known for many years that wild fruits and vegetables and their ancestors contain toxic substances. The levels of these natural toxins can be lowered by domestication and selective plant breeding.

Is America Ready for High-Tech Dining?

Genetic engineering has already made its way into medicine, producing drugs such as insulin, growth hormone, the clot-buster plasminogen activator, and other medicines such as vaccines for hepatitis B. Genetic engineering is also important in agriculture, making crops resistant to insects, diseases, and herbicides, producing foods that resist spoilage and have improved taste, texture, and nutritional value. By the end of the 20th century, 55% of the US crop of soybeans and 30% of the corn were genetically engineered. The FDA has approved genetically altered corn, summer squash, tomatoes, squash, and canola oil. Environmental activists have raised alarm over these foods, resulting in consumer concerns. Although there seems to be no direct scientific evidence that genetically engineered foods per se are dangerous, consumers nevertheless should be offered a choice between products that are genetically engineered and those that are not. Food labels should include this information.

One genetically engineered food that is clearly both nutritious and healthful is a genetically modified new grain, beta-carotene-enriched "golden rice." This product was scheduled in 2000 to become available, free of charge, to the developing countries of the world. This new strain contains high levels of yellow beta-carotene, which is a precursor to vitamin A. It was created by inserting genes from a daffodil and a bacterium into the rice genome. Widespread distribution of golden rice could prevent the majority of the 500,000 annual cases of blindness caused by vitamin A deficiency in developing countries.

What is genetic engineering? It is a process by which the DNA is removed from a plant and modified by inserting novel DNA representing a gene that contains the desired trait or traits. The modified DNA is then reintroduced into the plant. The recipient cells multiply and grow, expressing the new gene and displaying the new traits. This method is more selective and efficient than the traditional method of genetically modifying crops by selective breeding to develop strains that have higher yields, greater resistance to viruses, fungi, and insects, and superior color.

Choosing between natural and genetically modified foods and medicines

There is a bizarre asymmetry between the treatment and perception of natural organically grown foods, on the one hand, and those of genetically modified foods, on the other hand. There is no well-founded scientific evidence that genetically modified foods do any harm, yet there is furious opposition to such food, especially in Europe, where it is referred to as "Frankenfood." Contrast this status with that of a popular organic food, unpasteurized apple juice, which can sometimes be deadly because of bacterial contamination. Ancient farming methods are now being promoted in the West to produce expensive natural food without the use of possibly toxic agrochemicals. The affluent few who can afford these foods believe that if products are "natural," they must be safe and superior. At the same time, they decry genetically modified crops, which can be grown not only with less synthetic chemicals, but also more cheaply than conventional foods. The uninformed public's opposition to genetically modified products in the West is effectively killing development of the genetic-foods industry economically and thereby sentencing people in developing nations to food shortages and possible starvation.

A similar asymmetry exists between dietary supplements and modern pharmaceutical drugs. There is extensive evidence that unregulated dietary supplements can be dangerous if misused. Increasing numbers of Americans of all ages are falling ill or even dying after taking dietary supplements and herbal medicines (discussed in Chapter 3). Many of these people avoid the use of modern prescription drugs that have been designed to minimize side effects and to maximize beneficial treatment of a disorder.

Smoked Meats and Fish

Be cautious around the smoked meats. Is formaldehyde found in food? Yes, formaldehyde is in smoked meats and smoked fish, where it serves as a bactericide. It has been used as embalming fluid because it suppresses bacterial growth. As you probably have heard, formaldehyde is toxic; it is also a carcinogen. In the past, formaldehyde was used in bathroom deodorants. Cola and beer also contain small amounts of formaldehyde, 8 and 0.7 ppm (parts per million), respectively. Even your blood has some formaldehyde, 3 ppm, as the result of metabolism, but such tiny amounts of formaldehyde are not considered dangerous. In none of the above examples is formaldehyde considered toxic. This is an illustration that it is the *amount* of a toxic substance that must be considered when assessing risk. The smoking process by itself is insufficient to kill dangerous organisms in meat, as the following example demonstrates.

Beware of Jerky
(Trichinosis from Wild Game)

In 1955, a hunter in Idaho shot and killed a cougar. He proudly prepared homemade jerky with part of the meat—curing it in a salt brine solution he made from table salt of unknown salt concentration and then smoking the meat in a primitive smoke oven that did not generate a lot of heat. The hunter generously gave gift packages of the jerky to 14 of his friends. A few weeks later, after eating the meat, the hunter and 9 of his friends became ill with a fever, muscle aches, pain in the joints, fatigue, facial swelling, and a high blood count of white cells, suggesting a parasitic infection. Eventually, a diagnosis of trichinosis was made, an infection associated with the eating of raw or undercooked meat.

In the 1940s in the United States, about 500 cases of trichinosis were reported each year to the US Public Health Service. Because an unknown number of cases are not recognized and reported due to the usual mildness of the symptoms, the number of infected persons in those years was probably in the thousands. Pork is the number one source of the parasite. In recent years, however, the number of trichinosis cases from eating pork has been declining, while those resulting from consuming wild game meat have been increasing. From 1982 to 1986 in the United States, there were 69 known cases of trichinosis, with three deaths resulting from eating wild game meat. Consuming the flesh of bears accounted for 42 of the cases, wild pig meat accounted for 22, and the other 5 cases were from unidentified meat.

Over the past 25 years, three significant recorded endemics of trichinosis have occurred in Japan. In 1974, a group of hunters killed and ate raw meat from a black bear. Fifteen of the hunters developed clinical signs of trichinosis as described above. In 1980, several patrons of a Japanese restaurant ate the raw meat of a brown bear served as a delicacy; 12 persons were diagnosed with trichinosis. In 1982, raw black bear meat was served in a Japanese restaurant to 434 persons—60 subsequently were found to have trichinosis.

The parasite *Trichinella spiralis* can invade and reside in the muscles of any mammal; it has been found in mink, polar bears, tigers, sable, brown and black bears, walruses, raccoons, dogs, and several species of rodents. It is most commonly found in carnivorous and omnivorous animals that eat the meat of other animals, either killing them or acting as scavengers and eating the meat of dead animals. The deaths of three Swedish explorers were believed to have been caused by trichinosis from eating polar bear meat in 1897—their demise delayed the discovery of the North Pole by 12 years.

Since 1965, the Ministry of Health of Thailand has reported 5,400 cases of trichinosis, including 95 deaths. The sources of these infections have been hilltribe pigs (pigs raised like wild animals near villages) and wild boar. Pork dishes are delicacies in Thailand and are traditionally served on special occasions—the New Year, weddings, holidays, and any celebrations. The favorite dishes consist of finely chopped raw meat with local spices and hot chilies added.

Current trends are changing concerning the reservoirs and transmission of trichinosis; increasing numbers of wild animals are infected, and there are more infections of domestic animals, cattle, and sheep that accidentally eat or are fed meat or meat products infected with the parasite. In the United States, about 6% of ground beef products are contaminated with pork meat. Of the 90 million swine slaughtered in this country each year, about 100,000 carry the trichinosis parasite.

When a person eats meat infected with the parasite, the larvae are released from the meat by the action of digestive juices in the person's stomach. The larvae move into the small intestine, go through several developmental stages, become adults, and mate. Their newborn larvae migrate into the blood stream, travel throughout the body, and lodge in muscle tissue, often in the most active muscles of the body—the eye and chewing muscles, those of locomotion, and the heart, where invasion of the larvae may be fatal.

Freezing of meat will kill the larvae present, as will cooking it at 137 degrees Fahrenheit (58°C) or more for 10 minutes. A lesson to be learned here is that the eating of raw or undercooked meat is never advisable; as a health precaution, cook your meat. These interesting examples were found in Orlando Soave's *The Animal–Human Bond*, 2nd ed., San Francisco/Maryland: Austin Windield.

Alcoholic Beverages

Adults can buy alcoholic beverages in most grocery stores. What the world calls alcohol is actually ethyl alcohol, or ethanol; since antiquity, alcohol has been used and abused in socially acceptable, intoxicating beverages. Alcohol occurs naturally in our bodies, but in such small amounts that it has no physiological effect. If alcohol were to be discovered today, its sale would be forbidden because of its potentially lethal side effects. The use of alcohol, however, is deeply embedded in our society.

Physiologically, alcohol acts as a depressant. Like a general anesthetic, it acts to "freeze" the brain's cortex from inhibitory controls. Alcohol indirectly affects how the nerve cells work by enhancing the binding of the natural neurotransmitter GABA (gamma-aminobutyric acid). Certain tranquilizers and sedatives act in a similar way, and there is strong synergy between alcohol and these drugs. Valium can be lethal when taken with alcohol. The combination of phenobarbital, a sedative, and alcohol was used in the mass suicide of a cult in Rancho Santa Fe, California, in 1997. This is our first example of a common medical problem: particular combinations of otherwise useful drugs or physiologically active substances can be extremely dangerous. Such combinations are termed contraindicated.

Ethyl alcohol interferes with an antidiuretic hormone, leading to more frequent urination and eventually dehydration. It causes blood vessels to dilate; recall the red hue of a drinker or your own apparent feeling of warmth. In reality, a vasodilator causes a person to lose heat rather than to retain it; nevertheless, the myth persists that alcohol warms you when you are chilled.

Specific risks associated with women consuming alcohol were revealed by a 1998 analysis of six long-term studies on a total of more than 300,000 women. There is an increased risk of developing breast cancer, but the increase in risk is very small for those who consume no more than the equivalent of one glass of wine a day. If a woman drinks one glass a day, her chances of developing breast cancer would increase from 12.5% for a teetotaler to 13.6% over a lifetime of 85 years. This slight increase must be balanced against alcohol's benefit to the heart. Epidemiologic studies indicate that imbibing small quantities of ethyl alcohol reduces the incidence of heart disease. Each year, 500,000 women in the United States die of heart disease, compared with 43,000 who die of breast cancer. Whether or not to drink alcohol becomes a matter of individual choice. The underlying mechanism may be associated with the fact that alcohol raises the level of the female hormone estrogen, which is known to stimulate breast cancer growth.

A 1996 study showed that even modest amounts of alcohol raise the levels of estrogen in postmenopausal women who are taking oral estrogen as a therapy against heart disease and osteoporosis. The increased blood levels of estrogen induced by drinking even a glass of wine combined with oral estrogen therapy consequently might increase a woman's risk of breast cancer. Previous studies also have shown that alcoholic men also have elevated levels of estrogen.

Alcohol is made naturally by fermentation of carbohydrates and industrially by the reaction of water with gaseous ethylene. Despite the fact that these two products are chemically identical, alcoholic beverages are never manufactured from ethylene; even the Soviets, in a time of potato crop failure, would purchase only alcohol made by fermentation. This is an example of the illogical distinction between a natural versus a synthetic chemical.

Even birds, bees, and larger animals have trouble with alcohol consumption. They imbibe alcohol that occurs naturally in fermented sugar in the nectar of flowering plants, especially in hot weather, which promotes fermentation. Honeybees that drink fermented nectar have flying accidents, die younger, and are sometimes rejected by the teetotalers back at the hive. Honey can also become fermented in warm, humid conditions. It is suspected that alcohol-laced honey was the inspiration for the ancient alcoholic beverage mead. It has even been claimed that elephants in the Kruger National Park (Africa) get "stoned" on alcohol produced in their own stomachs. After the elephants eat fruit of the marula tree, drink copious amounts of water, and jog about, fermentation takes place. The alcohol produced in their own digestive vats sets these pachyderms galloping about with no reported harm to themselves.

The alcohol content of beer is up to 10% and that of wine up to 20%; above that level, the yeast cells carrying out fermentation die. For this reason, stronger drinks must be made by distillation: brandy (from wine), whiskey (from corn and other grains), vodka (from grains), and sake (from rice). In the United States, the alcohol content is denoted by "proof," which is equal to twice the percent alcohol (e.g., 100 proof is equivalent to 50% alcohol). At concentrations above 50%, alcohol can be lethal; pure, undiluted alcohol is lethal.

Beer is an ancient food. It was first fermented from grain about 3,500 years ago, about 2,000 years before grain was used to make bread. Until 300 years ago, it was safer to drink beer than to drink surface water because the water used in brewing had been boiled and thus disinfected. Beer is nearly a complete food. It contains water, carbohydrates, proteins, and nutrients such as the water-soluble B vitamins, including significant amounts of folic acid but no biologically active vitamin B_{12}. Beer does not contain any fat, and it has virtually none of the potentially toxic metals, such as cadmium, chromium, cobalt, lead, mercury, or tin. There is some evidence, however, that beer can be contaminated with the toxic element arsenic if the hops from which the beer is brewed are grown on arsenic-contaminated soil. Because most beers are isotonic (meaning they have the same osmotic pressure as body fluids), they have little effect on the water balance of the body. The modest levels of alcohol in beer reduce the risk of heart disease for light drinkers compared with heavy drinkers or abstainers.

Certain expensive alcoholic beverages may contain additional, possibly carcinogenic, chemicals called polycyclic aromatic hydrocarbons (PAHs). These compounds are present in all whiskey brands; Scotch malts are the worst offenders because these PAHs derive from the smoky peat used to introduce the special flavor to single-malt Scotch whiskey, the drink most favored by your author! Curiously, the similar Irish whiskey has much lower concentrations of PAHs. Whiskey drinkers are known to be more likely to develop bowel, mouth, and throat cancers, but the tiny amounts of PAHs present are not thought to be responsible for the higher rates of cancer in whiskey drinkers.

Other alcoholic beverages contain toxic substances. An interesting example is the emerald-green liqueur absinthe, derived from wormwood. Some say that addiction to absinthe drove the painter Vincent Van Gogh to take his own life. Other famous artists, Henri de Toulouse-Latrec and Pablo Picasso, painted absinthe drinkers, illustrating its popularity and dark side. It had long been recognized that absinthe can cause convulsions, hallucinations, and psychotic behavior. Many years ago, absinthe was very popular in Europe and in the United States, but it was banned in the period between 1905 and 1915. The toxic ingredient in absinthe, alpha-thujone, has been shown to block the brain's receptors for gamma-aminobutyric acid, or GABA, a natural inhibitor of nerve impulses. When GABA is blocked, neurons fire too easily and brain signals go out of control. One can still buy herbal preparations of this toxic, natural substance on the internet in the form of wormwood oil. In some countries, notably the Czech Republic, absinthe is available in a dilute, less potent form. Old absinthe contained about 260 parts per million of alpha-thujone, but the present-day drink has less than 10 parts per million.

How does our body rid itself of alcohol? This detoxification is carried out by a zinc enzyme in the liver, alcohol dehydrogenase; the product is a toxic chemical, acetaldehyde. This zinc enzyme is present because bacteria produce some alcohol in our body from carbohydrates, especially in our intestines. Even teetotalers have some alcohol in their body! The further metabolic transformation of acetaldehyde involves a second enzyme-catalyzed transformation to acetic acid. If this enzyme, acetaldehyde dehydrogenase, is impaired or inhibited, toxic acetaldehyde builds up. The drug Antabuse, an inhibitor of this second enzyme, has been used to help treat alcoholism. A patient taking Antabuse becomes ill whenever he or she drinks alcohol. Some common food additives or over-the-counter medications contain alcohol—for instance, vanilla extract (35% alcohol) and mouthwashes (Listerine is 25% alcohol). People taking Antabuse must be aware of the potential effects of using these products; they may become ill.

The two enzymes alcohol and acetaldehyde dehydrogenases are important factors in the complex diseases referred to as alcoholism. One manifestation of alcoholism is a low concentration of one or both of these enzymes, but many other factors are involved. In the United States, it affects about 2 people in 1,000; a higher percentage of women are alcoholics than men. On average, women do not metabolize alcohol as rapidly as men do, even when differences in body weight are taken into account. Some scientists believe this difference stems from moderately different levels of the two enzymes that detoxify alcohol. Some alcoholics have the capacity to metabolize large quantities of alcohol.

Susceptibility to alcoholism is thought to be at least partly genetic. A high incidence of alcoholism is observed among Native Americans and the bushmen of South Africa. This is further evidence that some alcoholism has a genetic origin. The gene (or genes) involved in inherited examples of alcoholism has not yet been identified, however.

Certain people of Asian origin are thought to lack the second enzyme, acetaldehyde dehydrogenase. The buildup of the toxic chemical acetaldehyde may account for their sudden flushing after consuming alcoholic beverages.

Alcohol dehydrogenase causes additional problems; it is a "promiscuous" enzyme in the sense that it also transforms alcohols other than ethyl alcohol, although not as efficiently. The smallest alcohol, methyl alcohol, is highly toxic for just this reason. Alcohol dehydrogenase transforms methanol into the toxic molecule formaldehyde. Formaldehyde damages not only the liver but also the eyes, where there is a small amount of alcohol dehydrogenase and another oxidizing enzyme, catalase. In some cases, blindness can result. It is interesting that one treatment for methyl alcohol poisoning is to drink large, intoxicating amounts of ethyl alcohol; the latter binds to the enzyme 20 times more strongly, thus inhibiting the unwanted oxidation of methyl alcohol, which is then passed through the kidneys and excreted in urine. This lock-and-key effect of enzyme specificity for a substrate (in this case ethyl alcohol) is a common property of enzymes. The popular artificial sweetener, NutraSweet, is a methyl ester of a dipeptide and will break down in the body, releasing methyl alcohol. Does this pose a risk? Probably not, since the amount of methyl alcohol released is about the same as we would get from consuming a glass of fruit juice, beer, or wine. Again, we find it is the *amount* of a chemical that is important in determining its toxicity.

Ethylene glycol, the active ingredient in antifreeze, is also converted into toxic substances in the body by the action of alcohol dehydrogenase. How would ethylene glycol get into your body, anyway? In the 1980s, some Italian wine manufacturers adulterated red wine with ethylene glycol because it is sweet (but poisonous). These criminals actually used an industrial solvent, diethylene glycol, because they did not understand nomenclature. Both compounds are toxic.

HERMAN®

by Jim Unger

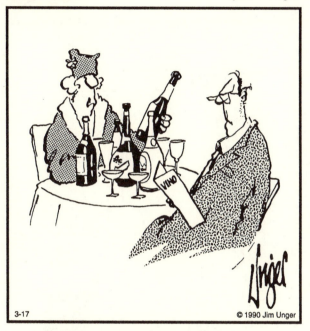

3-17

© 1990 Jim Unger

"I think you ordered us a three-course meal from the wine list."

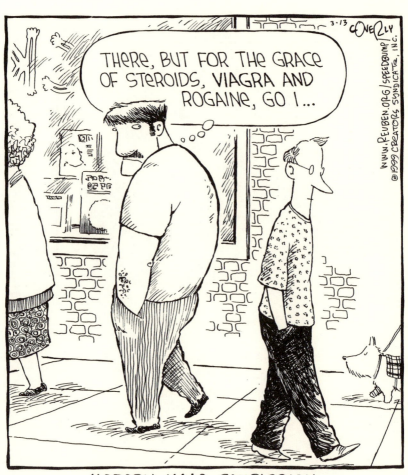

MODERN MALE COMPASSION

2

The Pharmacy

THE PHARMACY IS FILLED with toxic chemicals, but when properly used, these drugs are essential to our health. Some drugs are derived from natural substances; others are entirely synthetic. In the United States, all drugs, prescription and over-the-counter alike, are manufactured under rigorous control by the Food and Drug Administration. In this important sense, the pharmacy differs from the health-food store.

Prescription Drugs

Modern prescription drugs are powerful; they can be efficacious, but if the dose is too large or if the drug is taken with another, contraindicated medicine or food, these pharmaceuticals can be dangerous. Some knowledge of the way modern drugs work may help you understand their possible dangers.

Enzymes are biological catalysts that control the rates of reactions necessary for the function of all biological organisms from animals such as humans to bacteria. As in a fine watch, the transformations in a living organism must be properly timed to maintain a healthy state. In 1946, the famous chemist Linus Pauling proposed that compounds that inhibit or interfere with enzymes could act as drugs. In fact, many drugs, from ancient herbal medicines to modern designed pharmaceuticals, are enzyme inhibitors. For example, penicillin acts by destroying an enzyme that bacteria need to construct their cell walls. But penicillin and older drugs were discovered by accident rather than by design. Because modern recombinant DNA technology can be used to manufacture substantial amounts of any protein, scientists can unravel the structures and mechanism of action of the special proteins called enzymes. Armed with this knowledge, scientists are now able to design excellent drug candidates.

Research on enzyme inhibitors is leading to many useful drugs such as the "statins" (e.g., Mevacor, Pravachol, and Lipitor). These reversible enzyme inhibitors slow the biological synthesis of cholesterol. The new cholesterol-lowering statins work by inhibiting a major enzyme involved in synthesizing cholesterol in the liver. In individuals with high levels of serum cholesterol, as much as a 30% reduction in LDL, the "bad" cholesterol, can be achieved without reducing the "good" cholesterol, HDL. Five percent of the adult US population— some 9 million people—now take cholesterol-lowering drugs in the hope of warding off heart disease. Although these drugs significantly reduce the risk of dying of heart attacks, they have unexpected mental side effects: they may impair dexterity and attention. Speculation is that lowering cholesterol might also reduce needed brain chemicals. This possible side effect might result in a slight decrease in alertness or coordination that could be hazardous during activities like driving. The benefits of these cholesterol-lowering drugs are nevertheless considered to outweigh any possible risks.

The most familiar over-the-counter drug, aspirin, is also an enzyme inhibitor. The natural precursor of aspirin was first described in 400 B.C. by Hippocrates, the father of modern medicine. He used an infusion of willow bark to treat people with headaches and labor pains. Not until 23 centuries later, in 1899, however, did chemists isolate and modify the active ingredient of this remarkable drug, which also eases inflammation, reduces fevers, and even reduces the risk of heart disease. In 1971, Nobel laureate John Vane proposed that aspirin is an irreversible enzyme inhibitor. It is now known that both aspirin and popular, related drugs such as ibuprofen (e.g., Motrin) and naproxen (e.g., Aleve, Naprosyn), which are collectively referred to as nonsteroidal antiinflammatory drugs (NSAIDs), act in a similar way. These drugs, which have a worldwide market worth more than $9 billion a year ($8 billion in the United States), inhibit enzymes called cyclooxygenases, or COX, which catalyze the production of a group of fatty acids known as prostaglandins. The latter are hormones that play a variety of roles in the body by dilating veins, increasing the sensitivity of pain receptors on nerve endings, and inhibiting the immune system. More than one cyclooxygenase enzyme is involved, and the selective inhibition of different cy-clooxygenases may explain the diverse side effects of various members of this class of drugs.

Aspirin and similar NSAIDs are some of the most heavily used drugs in the world. NSAIDs are prescribed for a wide range of ailments, from fevers to migraine headaches and tennis elbows. There is a downside to NSAIDs. In some individuals, these drugs have serious side effects: stomach bleeding, ringing in the ears, dizziness, and nausea. This dilemma has been resolved by the discovery that there are two kinds of COX enzymes. One enzyme produces the "housekeeper" prostaglandins at modest levels to keep our stomach, blood platelets, kidneys, and other tissues in working order. The second COX enzyme is naturally produced only in times of trauma and generates high levels of the prostaglandins that cause inflammation. These COX-1 and COX-2 enzymes have been compared to a garden sprinkler and a water cannon, respectively. A new NSAID has been developed that blocks COX-2 and leaves COX-1 unaffected, thus controlling inflammation without disturbing our normal physiology. This "superaspirin," celecoxib (marketed as Celebrex), was developed by Monsanto and approved by the FDA in January, 1999. Another COX-2 inhibitor, rofecoxib (Vioxx), was released by the Merck pharmaceutical company six months later. These two medicines have become blockbuster drugs. They may have other uses in addition to relief of inflammation. For example, they may lower the incidence of colon and other cancers because aspirin and ibuprofen appear to reduce the incidence of some types of colon cancer. Some researchers have suggested that an aspirin a day may cut the risk of colon cancer in half!

The chemical structures of most synthetic drugs have one or more handed, or chiral, centers; thus, they are handed molecules that exist in two opposite, mirror-image forms. As in shaking hands with another person or putting on gloves, the interaction of mirror-image drugs with handed biological molecules is specific and necessarily different for the two forms. Typically, one handed form of a drug is efficacious, whereas the other is not and often exhibits dangerous side effects. In the manufacture of pharmaceutical drugs, huge sums of money are spent to isolate and sell only the efficacious handed form, which is the only form the FDA will usually allow to be sold. In 1996, the US market for chiral drugs was approximately $35 billion per year! This was not always so; mixtures of both handed forms of drugs were once sold and administered. For example, an infamous drug, thalidomide, was developed in Germany in the 1950s as a sedative to alleviate nausea during pregnancy. This drug was later found to have a terrible side effect connected to one of its handed forms. In 1961, it was found to produce fetal limb abnormalities during the first three months of pregnancy. Many tragic births of deformed infants resulted before this drug was withdrawn from the market. In the United States, the FDA came close to approving the drug but never did.

The tragedy with thalidomide had one good effect; thereafter, many governments—especially the United States—have required that only the single, efficacious handed form of a drug could be used. However, this restriction does not apply retroactively to the older, approved drugs. A case in point is the drug methylphenidate hydrochloride (trade name Ritalin), taken by an estimated 2 million children with attention deficit–hyperactivity disorder. Ritalin is still made and sold as an equal mixture of two mirror-image forms, called a racemate. Because of this, half of every Ritalin dose may contribute nothing to its therapeutic effect, while possibly adding to its side effects. Positron emission tomography studies of volunteers taking the drug revealed that there were significant differences in the way the two mirror image forms interacted with the brain. The efficacious form bound with dramatic specificity to the part of the brain, the basal ganglia, involved in the drug's therapeutic effect. It has been proposed that the other mirror form may contribute to Ritalin's side effects including insomnia and loss of appetite or to long-term complications such as liver damage.

Any physiologically active agent such as a pharmaceutical drug, either prescription or over-the-counter, will have maximum therapeutic dose limits. These doses are always marked on the container. A precaution in taking any drug has to do with its toxic side effects, which run parallel to the desired activity of the drug. This relationship is expressed as the therapeutic index (the ratio of toxicity to effectiveness). Unwanted side effects include upsetting the biological balance, or homeostasis, of the body's systems. The term *homeostasis* refers to the normal physiological equilibrium balance. For every biological action, there is an opposing reaction. A paramount example is the balance between the opposing actions of a vasodilator such as nitric oxide and a vasoconstrictor such as adrenaline. Many drugs act to restore balance to a biological system that is out of balance, but other drugs that would appear to be beneficial may actually upset this balance.

Contraindicated Drug Combinations

Because of this physiological balance, some drug combinations are contraindicated. The physiological activities of contraindicated drugs clash, creating a dangerous situation. The combination of amphetamines and alcohol is but one of many examples. Unfortunately, this problem is not uncommon when physicians, in haste or ignorance, prescribe a drug for a patient who is taking another, contraindicated medication, or the patient fails to inform the physician of his or her current medication. There are computer programs that can identify this problem, but such programs are not in general use. Your pharmacist, it is hoped, will warn you about such problems. Individuals are well advised to verify for themselves the use, proper dose, and possible drug interactions of their medications. I consult *The Johns Hopkins Handbook of Drugs* (Margolis, S., ed. 1993. New York: Random House), which emphasizes such problems for people past age 50.

Sometimes a previously unknown dangerous combination is discovered in routine clinical practice, with deadly results. A case in point is fen/phen, the combination of appetite suppressants fenfluramine and phentermine that in the late 1990s became the diet pill of choice among weight-conscious Americans. These two prescription drugs were tested and approved separately more than 20 years ago by the FDA, which later gave its blessing to their combined use. More than 18 million fen/phen prescriptions were written in 1996. Physicians at the Mayo Clinic in Minnesota and the Merit-Care Medical Center in North Dakota found that more than 20 patients who were using fen/phen had developed a heart-valve problem. The Mayo Clinic put out a public alert, warning of possible complications from this apparently synergistic drug combination. Fen/phen was taken off the market and became the subject of major lawsuits.

Other combinations of contraindicated drugs can be lethal. A deadly mixture is the new male-potency drug sildenafil citrate, trade name Viagra, taken with the illicit drugs known as "poppers" and methamphetamine. Soon after the introduction of Viagra, this combination killed several nightclub patrons in Hollywood. The victims took methamphetamine to get a "high" and then Viagra to restore the sexual potency that the methamphetamine takes away. In addition, they snorted "poppers" to enhance their sexual experience. Poppers are a combination of amyl nitrite, a prescription drug, and butyl ni-

threatening his leg with gangrene and certain amputation. The new drug penicillin was administered, and the infection soon abated. But then the pharmacy ran out of penicillin, and this unfortunate person died of his wound infection. My father would have died of a streptococcus infection except for this new miracle drug. Many of you would not be alive to read this book without the development of antibiotics.

Like all drugs, antibiotics are not entirely safe. Most antibiotic drugs can cause nausea, diarrhea, or a rash. Some of these adverse side effects result from the fact that antibiotic drugs also kill useful bacteria that occur naturally in the body. Sometimes fungi grow in the place of the natural bacteria, resulting in oral, intestinal, or vaginal *candidiasis* (thrush). In addition, some individuals experience a severe allergic reaction to an antibiotic, causing facial swelling, itching, or breathing difficulty. These people cannot take that particular antibiotic drug for the rest of their lives, because each new allergic reaction will become more severe.

Antibiotic drugs can also have unanticipated effects. Medical researchers have suspected that bacterial infections can cause heart disease. It has long been known that streptococcus ("strep") bacterial infections can damage the heart in the disease called rheumatic fever. That condition is rare, now that antibiotics are readily available. Nevertheless, at present, as many as 20% of heart-attack victims do not have any of the known risk factors for heart disease. In 1999, evidence was reported that a commonly occurring microorganism, chlamydia, produces a protein identical to one found in healthy heart tissue. In mouse studies, the mouse's immune system was found to attack this microorganism and thereby damage the heart and coronary arteries, which contained the same protein. Perhaps an immune response to chlamydiae is responsible for at least some of the 961,000 deaths that occur from heart attacks each year in the United States. This interesting hypothesis remains to be tested in large-scale human trials. If this hypothesis proves to be true, what could be done to control this additional risk factor? Taking antibiotics prophylactically is probably unwise, because chlamydiae would eventually become resistant, creating an even more serious problem. Immunization against chlamydia and related microbes might be the answer.

The Pharmacy

Over-the-Counter Medications

Over-the-counter drugs can be purchased without a doctor's prescription. Most of them are very old medications from the times before prescriptions drugs and are considered safe to be used without a doctor's supervision. Nevertheless, just like prescription drugs, over-the-counter medicines can be potent and can have deleterious side effects. The dose must be controlled, and there may be contraindicated combinations with other medicines, including herbal remedies.

Millions of Americans take nonsteroidal antiinflammatory drugs (NSAIDs) such as ibuprofen, naproxen, piroxicam, and aspirin. NSAIDs can promote bleeding ulcers in about 1% to 2% of people who take high doses. These ulcers are thought to result in 7,600 deaths in the United States each year. Similarly, overdosing on nonaspirin painkillers such as Tylenol can damage the liver. The active ingredient in Tylenol is acetaminophen. Even small amounts of acetaminophen may have a deleterious effect when taken by people who have not eaten for a prolonged period or who are heavy users of alcohol. As long as label instructions are carefully followed, acetaminophen is a perfectly safe and effective pain reliever for most people. Children should not be given aspirin, because it has been linked with Reye's syndrome, a potentially deadly disorder in children who take aspirin when they have flu or chickenpox, both of which may initially resemble a cold. This warning is better known in the United States, where it is placed on aspirin bottles, than it is in parts of Europe.

Medicines and Drugs Derived from Plants

This section describes medicinal products that are usually *not* found in present-day pharmacies or health-food stores. These powerful substances are derived from plants; some are legal, and others are not. These substances are all natural and might be considered herbal medicines except for legal restraints. One hundred years ago, these medicines would have been found in pharmacies. In some examples, chemists have modified these plant-derived natural drugs to make more potent compounds. I will start with drugs that dull the mind.

Marijuana (cannabis)

This natural drug has an ancient history. Marijuana, also called cannabis, is the most widely disseminated hallucinogenic drug in the world. Its source is the hemp plant, which was cultivated for fiber in northeastern China as early as 4000 B.C. Some believe that the Chinese used cannabis as a sedative as early as 2700 B.C. By 800 B.C., this hallucinogen had spread to India, where it was used in religious rites and as a medicine, even among common people. The cultivation and medical use of cannabis extended further to Persia and reached the entire Mediterranean by at least 300 A.D. The Muslim Arabs used this drug freely; cannabis is not forbidden in the Koran, even though alcohol is.

The mind-altering compound in hemp is tetrahydrocannabinol (THC), which is concentrated in a resin mostly in the flowers of the female plants. Different preparations of marijuana vary greatly in potency. Marijuana cigarettes, "joints," contain much more tar than tobacco cigarettes do and undoubtedly subject the smoker to even greater risks from the smoke and tar, but this topic has been little studied. This illicit smoke has a more pronounced odor than tobacco smoke does; your author has such a keen nose that I thought of retiring to become a "marijuana police dog" but decided against that occupation because of the poor working conditions.

In 1996, Arizona and California passed referenda that legalized the use of marijuana for persons suffering from cancer and AIDS to reduce pain and relieve nausea from chemotherapy. This treatment has not been approved by the FDA. In Britain, extracts from cannabis have been proposed for treatment of multiple sclerosis, glaucoma, and bronchial asthma. If the active agent, THC, were to be used as a pharmaceutical, there would be problems. THC has a narrow therapeutic window, and the side effects (dizziness, sedation, dry mouth, disconnected thought, and impaired memory) could rule out its use at high doses. Further, it would be unwise to administer psychotropic cannabiloids to patients with heart disease or schizophrenia.

The psychoactive effects of cannabis are slow to develop but are long lasting. Inhibition of both short- and long-term memory and

The Pharmacy

other cognitive functions result from THC binding to and retention in specific neural membranes of the brain. In contrast to human susceptibility to opiates, there are few THC receptors in the brainstem, which controls pulse and respiration. One therefore cannot get "stoned" to death; however, there is danger in driving or operating heavy machinery while under the influence of THC. Several serious train accidents have been linked to the operators' use of marijuana.

Marijuana is not regarded as particularly dangerous by many members of the American public; approximately 24 million Americans had tried this drug in 1972. In 1996, the use of cannabis rose again, especially among youth. Marijuana is sometimes cited as the bridge young people cross on their way to harder (more potent) drugs such as heroin and cocaine.

Hemp for illegal marijuana production is said to be the major cash crop in some southern states. Several strains of cannabis grown for fiber (industrial hemp) are low in THC and are of no interest for either recreational or medical use. Nevertheless, many law-enforcement agencies oppose the commercial cultivation of industrial hemp because of complications over enforcement of drug statutes.

Opium

Probably the oldest drug, opium is obtained from the opium poppy (Figure 5, see color section). Opium has been used, perhaps for thousands of years, to relieve pain and alter consciousness. There is indirect evidence that opium was used as long ago as 4000 B.C. in shallow lake villages in what is now Switzerland. It is certain that, by 1500 B.C., opium was used in the eastern Mediterranean. Ancient recipes for preparing opium from poppies show that opium was a well-established painkiller and was used for religious ceremonies— what a way to attract a congregation! For many centuries, opium was a legitimate, uncontrolled drug. Until 1906, with passage of the Pure Food and Drug Act, *no drugs were restricted* in the United States. In the 19th century, anyone in the United States could buy opium in a general store. Myriad patent medicines were peddled from wagons in the American West; many were laced with opium (as well as with alcohol, especially for those who otherwise "abstained"). Such practices were not confined to the United States. In the 1800s, opium was a fashionable social drug in England, where more than 60,000 pounds were consumed each year.

Morphine

The active ingredient in opium is morphine. Morphine is used to alleviate severe, chronic pain, particularly in cancer patients. Some patients suffering from chronic pain can return to normal lives when their pain is controlled by morphine. Some physicians believe morphine has been and continues to be underutilized. Why? The problem is the association of morphine with its cousin, heroin, a synthetic derivative that is converted back to morphine in the body.

Heroin

Morphine and heroin have similar structures. Heroin is an illegal street drug. Both substances are addictive, but heroin is much more so. A 1980 study showed that in a hospital setting, only 0.03% of 11,882 patients became addicted to morphine, whereas 10% to 30% of the people who try heroin become addicted. Morphine produces much less euphoria than heroin. Heroin withdrawal is said to feel like a violent flu. Of course, both drugs have side effects, but heroin's are more dramatic. For example, heroin dulls libido in both men and women by suppressing the brain's output of sex hormones. The different potencies have to do with the different rates that these drugs pass through the blood–brain barrier.

Codeine

The painkiller codeine is natural; it occurs in small amounts in opium. The structure of codeine differs from that of morphine by an additional carbon atom on codeine. Codeine, which is manufactured by modifying morphine, is a strong analgesic. For example, mixed with acetaminophen, codeine is used to reduce pain during kidney stone episodes or after tooth extractions. It is also used in some prescription cough medicines. Although codeine is also somewhat addictive, it is much more widely used and accepted than morphine.

Cocaine

The Spanish Conquistadors discovered another plant-derived native medicine that was very much in the news in the 1990s: cocaine. The Incas chewed the leaves of the coca plant as a stimulant and analgesic; native peoples in the high Andes still do this today, at the rate of about 13 million pounds per year.

The Spanish conquerors encouraged the Incas, who were pressed into work in gold mines, to use cocaine. No wonder—this drug suppresses hunger and helps the user sustain heavy manual labor! Although not documented, cocaine was widely said to have been used in a popular American beverage at the beginning of the 1900s, thus the name Coca Cola (which does not contain this ingredient now). Currently, large quantities of cocaine are manufactured in clandestine laboratories in South America; the neutral compound, known as "free-base" cocaine, and the hydrochloride salt, called "crack" cocaine, are shipped to the United States and Europe. As an illicit recreational drug, cocaine has been responsible for a major crime problem across the United States. The free-base form is inhaled (snorted) as a powder; crack cocaine is smoked (a more dangerous method). For various reasons, the more dangerous use of crack cocaine carries much greater federal penalties, an issue that is politically charged.

Synthetic narcotics

Synthetic modifications of naturally occurring narcotic drugs are made by chemically tacking on or snipping off an atom or two. The resultant drug can be extremely potent and very difficult to detect, and it may even be legal until a new law is devised banning each new modification. Some new "designer drugs" began in California (where else?) and have been spreading to the rest of the country. One example is a compound known as MPPP, which is structurally identical to the prescription analgesic meperidine hydrochloride (Demerol), except that one carbon and one oxygen atom are switched. MPPP is said to produce effects similar to those of heroin. An impurity in this illicit designer drug literally destroyed the brains of seven young addicts.

Designer drugs can be much more potent than their natural counterparts. It has been estimated that in one day, a single chemist could create enough artificial heroin to supply the entire nation's daily heroin demand. For example, a new variant, fentanyl, is 3,000 times more potent than heroin. You could kill 50 people with an amount that would fit on the head of a pin! If such a synthetic narcotic was not diluted at least one-hundred-fold, a user could easily take a lethal overdose. Such uncontrolled drugs have probably killed many users. These drugs cannot be detected in routine urine tests such as those given prisoners! You can understand the attraction of the designer drug business to criminals. From an investment of $1,500 in equipment, millions of dollars in profit can be made.

Quinine

Derived from the bark of a South American "fever tree," quinine was discovered by Peruvian Indians and adopted by the conquering Spanish. For more than 300 years, quinine was the only effective treatment for the mosquito-borne parasitic disease malaria. Quinine has a bitter taste because it is a base. Quinine bitters are still served with gin in gin-and-tonic drinks.

Malaria has been a scourge since antiquity. It played a crucial role in the defeat of the Athenian army at Syracuse in 413 B.C., was partially responsible for McClellan's defeat in the Chickahominy Valley of Virginia in 1862 and for the failure of the French to complete the Panama Canal at the turn of the 20th century, and it hastened the surrender of the American forces at Corregidor (now part of the Philippines) in 1942. Malaria is a problem in all tropical and semi-tropical areas. Because of fear of malaria, the marshland around San Francisco Bay was oiled to combat mosquitoes in the early 1900s. At the outbreak of World War II in the Pacific, the sole commercial source of quinine was in Java, Indonesia. As Indonesian plantations fell to the Japanese, the United States scrambled to discover and manufacture synthetic antimalarial drugs. The result was a new substitute for quinine, called chloroquine, along with a remarkable nontoxic insecticide called dichlorodiphenyl-trichloroethane (DDT), which reduced the incidence of malaria so United States forces could fight in the jungles of the Pacific. Later, this combination nearly defeated malaria, but unfortunately a drug-resistant, virulent form of malaria has surged in recent years. Malaria still infects 300 million people each year and kills 1.5 to 2.7 million!

Some other herbal drugs are effective against malaria, and for this reason, pharmaceutical companies continually scour reports of folk medicine, especially in Asia. A case in point is a traditional Chinese remedy, ginghaosa. The active compound in this herb, artemether, was found to be as effective as quinine in preventing malaria deaths. The need for an alternative to quinine has become urgent because of the developing quinine resistance of the mosquito-borne parasite. Of course, both drugs have side effects; quinine may cause low blood sugar, or hypoglycemia, and artemether may cause convulsions. Nothing so potent is risk free, even natural herbal medicines.

Taxol

Another drug extracted from a plant has been much in the news in the 1990s. This is paclitaxel (trade name Taxol), which has been touted as a potent anticancer drug used to treat both breast and ovarian cancers. Taxol is derived from the bark of the Pacific yew, a somewhat rare tree used by the northwestern American Indians in their folk medicine. The yew tree also has a special place in European history, the poisonous effects of its leaves noted in folklore. Yew wood was important in archery, and yew trees were often planted in churchyards so that the leaves would not be eaten by cattle, and there would be a plentiful supply of the wood to make bows.

Unfortunately, obtaining Taxol kills the yew tree, and the natural supply is not sufficient to allow for large-scale clinical use. The bark from two yew trees gives barely enough of the drug to treat a single cancer patient. There are two possible solutions to this dilemma: synthesize Taxol in the laboratory, or find an alternative natural source. Both have been done. A close chemical relative of Taxol can be obtained on a large scale from the needles of a European yew— without killing the tree. This substance can be converted readily into Taxol. This research has a bonus: another derivative of Taxol, taxerene, was prepared from the European yew and is a more potent anticancer drug. This is a relatively recent example of an old idea: modify and improve a naturally occurring drug through chemical carpentry.

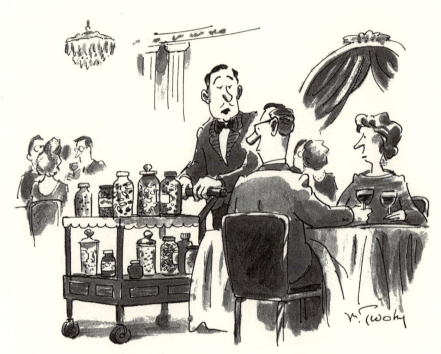

"Something from the supplement cart?"

3

Is "Health Food Store" an Oxymoron?

Herbal Medicines

Numerous herbs are taken as medicines to relieve particular ailments. Whereas many of these herbs may be harmless or even beneficial, others are potentially toxic. Just like synthetic drugs, herbs can be dangerous when taken in too-high doses or by people with contraindicated medical conditions. An example is the powerful herb foxglove, used in the late 1700s to treat congestive heart failure. It is still used for that purpose today. Two components in foxglove are presently used as heart medicine, but only by prescription. In higher doses, these natural chemicals can be dangerous.

Thousands of plant-derived substances (herbal extracts) and naturally occurring biochemicals can be purchased without prescription from health food stores and on the internet. Encyclopedias describing such herbs claim a variety of beneficial effects, but these claims are often based on flimsy data—very seldom on evidence from the double-blind studies required by the FDA before approving prescription drugs or most over-the-counter medicines.

This lack of control of health-food supplements has political roots: some powerful politicians are protective of natural remedies, which are popular with many voters. In 1994, Congress removed food supplements from FDA's jurisdiction. The Dietary Supplement Health and Education Act of 1994, sponsored by Senator Orrin Hatch (R-Utah), limits the federal government's regulation of dietary supplements. According to this act, herbal medicines are classified as supplements, not drugs. However, manufacturers are not permitted to say on labels that their herbal products prevent or treat specific diseases or symptoms.

In the United States, there is no monitoring of food-supplement quality control by a federal agency. The FDA warns that legal does not mean safe. These herbal preparations and natural biochemicals, such as minerals, vitamins, and hormones, are very seldom prepared using the strict manufacturing standards required for every medicine, either prescription or over-the-counter, sold in the drugstore. This situation is different in Germany, where herbal medicines have been more extensively studied and are regulated by the government. There, the growing, harvesting, and processing of herbal medicines are government controlled.

More than half of all Americans take herbs and dietary supplements, and at least 25% take them daily. As stated before, many people believe wrongly that if something is natural, it must be safe and is probably efficacious. A large portion of the adult population is increasingly turning to alternative medicines (mostly herbs) to alleviate or prevent symptoms from everyday ailments such as the common cold. In 1994, Americans spent about $1 billion on herbs and other tonics; if minerals and vitamins are included, the tally would be $4.6 billion. This loosely regulated industry sells products with often questionable safety and efficacy. Many patients do not tell their doctors they have been taking such products. They seek advice from magazines, the internet, and herbalists. But anyone can call himself or herself an herbalist and offer all kinds of advice, correct or not.

Are herbal medicines safe and efficacious? There is no single, simple answer to that question. It depends on the particular herb and its purity and concentration. Because herbs have been around for a long time and many have few or no side effects, the majority are not dangerous. The active ingredients in most herbal remedies are present in low concentrations. For this reason, herbs have been described as dilute drugs. Certain ones are dangerous and are prohibited in some European countries but are still sold in the United States.

Herbal medicines and home remedies have been used since the dawn of time. Indeed, many modern drugs such as paclitaxel (Taxol), which is used to treat breast and ovarian cancers, and ancient drugs—for example, willow bark tea, an ancient form of aspirin—were derived from plant products. Pharmaceutical companies are eager to test plant substances that are used in folk medicines. Not everything coming from plants is safe, however. Some of the most toxic substances known are plant products; Socrates was forced to commit suicide using hemlock, and strychnine has been used as a poison for centuries. There are legions of highly toxic plant products.

Nature has a huge chemical arsenal. Some naturally occurring products are important powerful drugs, others are deadly, but many are somewhere in between these extremes. In some cases, herbal drugs are effective. An herb from the plant called St. John's Wort, *Hypericum perforatum,* has been shown in European clinical studies to be effective in easing the symptoms of mild to moderate depression. This natural substance goes back 2,400 years in folk medicine; it appeals to many people, especially in Europe. St. John's Wort is the most widely used herbal supplement currently sold in Europe. In Germany, physicians write more than 3 million prescriptions a year for it—25 times the number they write for Prozac (fluoxetine hydrochloride). In 1997, Americans spent $1.7 billion on Prozac, making it the third biggest selling prescription drug in the country that year. The herb costs about $0.60 a day compared with Prozac at $2.50 or more daily. Both antidepressants raise the level of the "feel-good" brain chemical serotonin by inhibiting its uptake. Testing has yet to isolate the active ingredient or combination of ingredients in St. John's Wort. One component in St. John's Wort, a compound called hyperican, is toxic whenever the person taking this herb is exposed to sunlight. In the presence of hyperican, sunlight converts oxygen into a reactive form called singlet oxygen. This form produces painful skin lesions, a phenomenon long recognized by veterinarians. Cattle who graze on St. John's Wort in a sunny field develop facial lesions and severe loss of fur; a few cattle have died. Commercial bottles of this herbal medicine mention light sensitivity as a side effect. The chemical structure of Prozac is quite different from hyperican, and therefore does not have this photochemical side effect.

Doctors need to be told whether their patients have been taking St. John's Wort because this herb is reported to interfere with essential medications prescribed for people with AIDS and for organ-transplant recipients. This is an interesting example of contraindicated medicines in which one medicine is a prescription drug and the other is an uncontrolled herbal supplement. St. John's Wort is also contraindicated for patients taking antiseizure medication. Several violent seizures have been reported in epileptics within days of their initial use of St. John's Wort. These seizures ceased as soon as St. John's Wort was discontinued. On rare occasions, grand mal seizures have been observed in individuals with no prior history of seizure disorders soon after they took St. John's Wort.

Is "Health Food Store" an Oxymoron?

In 1999, St. John's Wort and two other popular herbal remedies were reported to have ill effects on human eggs and sperm; the other remedies are *Echinacea* species and *Ginkgo biloba.* These studies indicated a reduced ability of sperm to penetrate the egg and changes in the genetic material in the sperm, suggesting a potential risk to those who take these herbs. Another, more troubling finding, in the case of St. John's Wort, is a preliminary report of a mutation of the tumor-suppressor gene *BRCA1.* This mutation could possibly increase the risk of breast and ovarian cancers in women who inherit the mutated gene! Whether these herbs have adversely affected human health remains uncertain. If these were synthetic drugs, as opposed to natural drugs, however, such side effects probably would have prevented their release by the FDA.

One of the most frequently used remedies for the common cold is the herbal medicine mentioned above, *Echinacea* (pronounced ek-i-NAY-sha). This substance is derived from extracts of a plant from the daisy family. This herb has been used as a traditional medicine by Native Americans. A few controlled trials in humans have suggested that this extract may temporarily boost the body's immune system and increase resistance to respiratory infections. Some people may be allergic to this substance, and people with autoimmune diseases should use *Echinacea* with caution.

You may now understand why I usually defer when offered an "herbal tea." Let's look into a few more examples. A case in point is Herbal Ecstasy, widely advertised on the radio, in magazines, and on the internet. Similar products are sold under the names Cloud 9 and Ultimate Xphoria; these substances are touted as alternatives to illicit street drugs such as Ecstasy. The advertisements promise euphoria and heightened sexual feeling. The active ingredient, ephedrine, is in an herbal remedy, ma huang, that has been used in traditional Chinese medicine for centuries. These preparations, sometimes mixed with other herbs and chemicals, are touted as aids for losing weight, relieving respiratory ailments, and boosting energy. FDA scientists report serious adverse effects including heart attack, stroke, angina, and irregular heartbeats. These products have also been associated with seizures, psychiatric disorders, dizziness, personality changes, and memory loss. By 1996, at least 17 deaths were linked to these ephedrine preparations! The FDA may require warning labels and dose levels but unfortunately cannot ban sales!

If something is herbal, the public's misconception is that it is safe. Marketing of intoxicating herbs takes advantage of a gray area in FDA regulations; as mentioned, the 1994 law limits the agency's ability to regulate the sale of herbs and vitamins provided that no health claims are made. The burden is on the FDA to *prove* a preparation is not safe; for drugs in your pharmacy, the opposite standard applies. Because their physiological effects are not well understood and their purity is not guaranteed, herbs should never be given to babies or children except under medical supervision. Pregnant and breast-feeding women are advised not to take herbal products.

Poppy seeds contain morphine and codeine, and they have been used for centuries as a folk remedy. Poppy seeds remain a legal source of opiates, but with repeated use, they can produce high levels of morphine in the blood. Bakers occasionally have become addicted by occupational exposure to poppy seeds! Individuals who are subject to drug tests are well advised to avoid foods containing poppy seeds.

Some herbs that were widely available in health food stores are health hazards and have been taken off the market. An example is sassafras, the original flavoring in natural root beer. Sassafras contains a carcinogen, safrole, that was banned decades ago by the FDA from use in foods.

A substance derived from apricot and peach seeds, known as laetrile, has been touted as a cure or a preventative for cancer. The FDA believes laetrile is highly toxic because it can release cyanide. In fact, it may have caused the death of actor Steve McQueen, who died in 1980 after consuming laetrile in Mexico, where it is still sold in clinics as a cancer treatment. Several states have made laetrile legal as a nutritional supplement, and it can be purchased on the internet. Apricot kernels can be purchased as a source of laetrile across the United States in many health food stores. Laetrile sales are illegal only if it is sold as a cure for cancer. There is no double-blind study showing laetrile is efficacious, but it does contain a well-documented toxic substance.

Some Chinese herbs purchased in California have been found to be contaminated with poisonous elements such as lead, mercury, and arsenic. These impurities may have come from growing the herbs in polluted soil near industrial plants that spew out toxic wastes. Other Chinese herbal medicines derived from toads or insects are intrinsically toxic. For example, toad venom, or *bufonis venenum*, a secretion from the glands of certain toads, can affect heart muscles and cause paralysis and death. Some scorpion venoms, extracted from dried scorpions, are sometimes used to treat seizures and have deadly characteristics similar to venom from poisonous snakes.

Testosterone levels may explain the use of ground elk antlers by Koreans and Chinese who believe this product, used as a food supplement, reduces blood pressure, relieves arthritis, and improves male sexual performance. When cut off during the velvet stage, bull elk antlers are purportedly rich in the male sex hormone testosterone. There is apparently no serious scientific study of this folklore.

Sometimes herbal medicines and FDA-approved pharmaceutical drugs are one and the same. An example is a brick-red powder that comes from rice fermented with a red yeast. This substance has been used in China for 2,000 years as an herbal remedy and a food (a marinade for duck and pork). It seems to lower cholesterol levels. It should, because it contains lovastatin, the key component of a cholesterol-lowering prescription drug. This is a case in which "Foods are medicines; medicines are foods" as stated by Loren Israelson, a director at the Utah Natural Products Alliance. The US government may force this ancient food product off the market because of the dangers of the unregulated use of lovastatin.

Vitamins

What are vitamins and what do they do? Do we need to take vitamin supplements? Vitamins are natural organic molecules that some higher animals, including humans, need in small amounts. All forms of life use the same vitamins in their metabolism, but higher animals have lost the ability to make vitamins and so must obtain them by eating a balanced diet. Most vitamins are helper, or prosthetic, groups that are required by particular enzymes. Vitamins are usually categorized into those that are soluble in water and those that are soluble in fat. Because excesses of water-soluble vitamins are eliminated in the urine, these are rarely toxic.

Vitamins are constantly in the news. It has become "fashionable" to take additional vitamin supplements. In some situations, this supplementation is beneficial; in others, an excess dose of certain vitamins can be toxic (Table 3). In the 1990s, "vitamania" swept the United States. An estimated 100 million Americans spent over $4

Table 3 Human vitamin and mineral requirements, sources, functions, and symptoms of deficiency[a]

Vitamin	Major Dietary Sources	Functions in the Body	Possible Symptoms of Deficiency or Extreme Excess
WATER-SOLUBLE VITAMINS			
Vitamin B_1 (thiamine)	Pork, legumes, peanuts, whole grains	Coenzyme used in removing CO_2 from organic compounds	Beriberi (nerve disorders, emaciation, anemia)
Vitamin B_2 (riboflavin)	Dairy products, meats, enriched grains, vegetables	Component of coenzymes FAD and FMN	Skin lesions such as cracks at corners of mouth
Niacin	Nuts, meats, grains	Component of coenzymes NAD^+ and $NADP^+$	Skin and gastrointestinal lesions, nervous disorders. *Flushing of face and hands, liver damage*
Vitamin B_6 (pyridoxine)	Meats, vegetables, whole grains	Coenzyme used in amino acid metabolism	Irritability, convulsions, muscular twitching, anemia. *Unstable gait, numb feet, poor coordination*
Pantothenic acid	Most foods: meats, dairy products, whole grains, etc.	Component of coenzyme A	Fatigue, numbness, tingling of hands and feet
Folic acid (folacin)	Green vegetables, oranges, nuts, legumes, whole grains (also made by colon bacteria)	Coenzyme in nucleic acid and amino acid metabolism	Anemia, gastrointestinal problems. *May mask deficiency of vitamin B_{12}*
Vitamin B_{12}	Meats, eggs, dairy products	Coenzyme in nucleic acid metabolism; needed for maturation of red blood cells	Anemia; nervous system disorders

continued on next page

67

Table 3 Human vitamin and mineral requirements, sources, functions, and symptoms of deficiency
(continued)

Vitamin	*Major Dietary Sources*	*Functions in the Body*	*Possible Symptoms of Deficiency or Extreme Excess*
Biotin	Legumes, other vegetables	Coenzyme in synthesis of fat, meats	Scaly skin inflammation; neuromuscular disorders
Vitamin C (ascorbic acid)	Fruits and vegetables, especially citrus fruits, broccoli, cabbage, tomatoes, green peppers	Used in collagen synthesis (e.g., for bone, cartilage, gums); antioxidant; aids in detoxification; improves iron absorption	Scurvy (degeneration of skin, teeth, blood vessels), weakness, delayed wound healing, impaired immunity. *Gastrointestinal upset*
FAT-SOLUBLE VITAMINS			
Vitamin A (retinol)	Provitamin A (beta-carotene) in deep green and orange vegetables and fruits; retinol in dairy products	Component of visual pigments; needed for maintenance of epithelial tissues; antioxidant; helps prevent damage to lipids of cell membranes	Vision problems; dry, scaling skin. *Headache, irritability, vomiting, hair loss, blurred vision, liver and bone damage*
Vitamin D	Dairy products, egg yolk (also made in human skin in presence of sunlight)	Aids in absorption and use of calcium and phosphorus; promotes bone growth	Rickets (bone deformities) in children, bone softening in adults. *Brain, cardiovascular, and kidney damage*
Vitamin E (tocopherol)	Vegetable oils, nuts, seeds	Antioxidant; helps prevent damage to lipids of cell membranes	None well documented in humans; possibly anemia
Vitamin K (phylloquinone)	Green vegetables, tea (also made by colon bacteria)	Important in blood clotting	Defective blood clotting. *Liver damage and anemia*

Mineral[b]	Dietary Sources	Some Major Functions in the Body	Symptoms of Deficiency
Calcium (Ca)	Dairy products, dark green vegetables, legumes	Bone and tooth formation, blood clotting, nerve and muscle function	Retarded growth, possibly loss of bone mass
Phosphorus (P)	Dairy products, meats, grains	Bone and tooth formation, acid–base balance, nucleotide synthesis	Weakness, loss of minerals from bone, calcium loss
Sulfur (S)	Proteins from many sources	Component of certain amino acids	Symptoms of protein deficiency
Potassium (K)	Meats, dairy products, many fruits and vegetables, grains	Acid–base balance, water balance, nerve function	Muscular weakness, paralysis, nausea, heart failure
Chlorine (Cl)	Table salt	Acid–base balance, formation of gastric juice	Muscle cramps, reduced appetite
Sodium (Na)	Table salt	Acid–base balance, water balance, nerve function	Muscle cramps, reduced appetite
Magnesium (Mg)	Whole grains, green leafy vegetables	Cofactor; ATP bioenergetics	Nervous system disturbances
Iron (Fe)	Meats, eggs, legumes, whole grains, green leafy vegetables	Component of hemoglobin and of electron-carriers in energy metabolism; enzyme cofactor	Iron-deficiency anemia, weakness, impaired immunity
Fluorine (F)	Drinking water, tea, seafood	Maintenance of tooth (and probably bone) structure	Higher frequency of tooth decay

continued on next page

69

Table 3 Human vitamin and mineral requirements, sources, functions, and symptoms of deficiency
(continued)

Mineral[b]	Dietary Sources	Some Major Functions in the Body	Symptoms of Deficiency
Zinc (Zn)	Meats, seafood, grains	Component of certain digestive enzymes and other proteins	Growth failure, scaly skin inflammation, reproductive failure, impaired immunity
Copper (Cu)	Seafood, nuts, legumes, organ meats	Enzyme cofactor in iron metabolism, melanin synthesis, electron transport	Anemia, bone and cardiovascular changes
Manganese (Mn)	Nuts, grains, vegetables, fruits, tea	Enzyme cofactor	Abnormal bone and cartilage
Iodine (I)	Seafood, dairy products, iodized salt	Component of thyroid hormones	Goiter (enlarged thyroid)
Cobalt (Co)	Meats and dairy products	Component of vitamin B_{12}	None, except as B_{12} deficiency
Selenium (Se)	Seafood, meats, whole grains	Enzyme cofactor; antioxidant in close association with vitamin E	Muscle pain; possibly heart muscle deterioration
Chromium (Cr)	Brewer's yeast, liver, seafood, meats, some vegetables	Involved in glucose and energy metabolism	Impaired glucose metabolism
Molybdenum (Mo)	Legumes, grains, some vegetables	Enzyme cofactor	Disorder in excretion of nitrogen-containing compounds

[a]From Table 37.2, Campbell, N. A. 1997. *Biology*. Menlo Park, Calif.: Benjamin Cummings. pp. 814–15.
[b]All of these minerals are also harmful when consumed in excess.

billion each year on vitamin and mineral pills despite the absence of a scientific consensus as to whether taking vitamin supplements is valuable for people who eat relatively healthy diets. Even for individuals who may need more vitamins (smokers, the elderly, and pregnant women), the long-term benefits are unclear. Furthermore, because they are dietary supplements, vitamins are not subject to government testing for safety or purity.

Vitamins (and other nutrients) have to be absorbed by the body's cells in order to be used. If you depend on swallowing a pill to obtain the Recommended Dietary Allowance, RDA, of a particular vitamin, you should know that the amount actually absorbed, and therefore useful, is probably far less than what you could obtain by eating food. Taking megadoses or single supplements of multivitamins and minerals can be dangerous. Minerals can interfere with one another. A high dose of one can block the absorption of another. For example, high levels of iron in the diet can reduce zinc absorption. Zinc and copper also compete with one another. Fads can be dangerous. A few years ago, some nutritionists gave volunteers high doses of zinc. To their horror, the volunteers had heart attacks, although none was fatal. The zinc had apparently made them deficient in copper. It is better and safer to get the micronutrients you need from your diet.

There are other known dangers of vitamin use. High doses of vitamin E can interfere with the action of vitamin K, which is necessary for blood clotting. Large amounts of the mineral supplement calcium can limit the absorption of iron.

Vitamin C is well known to the general public. Following the suggestion of Linus Pauling, many people take one gram or more daily to fight off a cold, even though there is little evidence that this treatment has a positive effect. The other name for vitamin C, ascorbic acid, shows that it is an acid. Ascorbate, the ionized form of ascorbic acid, serves as an antioxidant. One of vitamin C's roles is in the synthesis of the connective protein collagen. A deficiency of vitamin C results in scurvy, which was a major medical problem among sailors in the 17th and 18th centuries. The skin lesions and weakened blood vessels associated with scurvy are the direct result of imperfect collagen. Supplementing the diet of seafarers with fresh vegetables or fruits solved this deficiency. Limes are rich in vitamin C and are effective in warding off scurvy; it is from this remedy that British sailors became known as "limeys."

If you do take vitamin C, buy it as ascorbic acid, which is the

Is "Health Food Store" an Oxymoron?

same thing only cheaper. How much vitamin C should you take? There is disagreement on that point. The conservative US Institute of Medicine recommends a daily allowance of 60 milligrams (an amount equal in size to about one-third of a standard aspirin tablet), but a study by the American biochemist Alfred Ordman proposes healthy adults take 500 milligrams twice a day. He has patented this dose, which is based upon the rate the body excretes vitamin C through the kidneys into the urine. If you go above 500 milligrams, you are just making expensive urine.

The water-soluble B vitamins are important components of enzymes called coenzymes. The very complex structure of vitamin B_{12} has a cobalt–carbon bond at its center. Several vital enzymes require vitamin B_{12} as a coenzyme; the cobalt atom is central to these chemical reactions. However, the detailed mechanisms of these B_{12}-catalyzed reactions are as yet poorly understood. The impaired absorption of the B_{12} cofactor results in pernicious anemia. This vitamin is made by anaerobic bacteria, but it makes its way into virtually all animal tissues. Animal products are the only dietary source of this vitamin; liver is an important source. Nutritional deficiency of vitamin B_{12} is rare except in strict vegetarians. However, perhaps 20% to 30% of the elderly have B_{12} deficiency resulting from atrophy of the stomach; they secrete less acid and so cannot break the vitamin off from proteins in the food. These people must obtain B_{12} through synthetic supplements, fortified cereals, or injections. The normal body requirement is tiny—0.01 milligram per day.

Eat green vegetables! Vitamin B_2, or folic acid, is found in Brussels sprouts, spinach, lettuce, and in many fruits, including apples and oranges. However, unlike most vitamins, the natural form of folic acid is not as easily absorbed by the body as are the synthetic forms found in vitamin supplements and fortified cereals. A deficiency in folic acid is responsible for a devastating, not uncommon birth defect called a neural tube defect, which develops in the first two weeks of pregnancy, long before most women realize they are pregnant. This problem can be prevented if the mother takes folic acid supplements within the first 6 weeks of pregnancy. This birth defect, which occurs in 1 in 1,000 babies, may stem from an aberrant gene that makes a less effective enzyme that uses folic acid as a cofactor; the enzyme needs more folic acid than normal to do its job. For this reason, all women who might become pregnant should take 400 IU (international units) of supplemental folic acid.

Is "Health Food Store" an Oxymoron?

Since January 1, 1998, breads, rice, and pasta have been fortified with folic acid, which will probably have the beneficial effect of lowering homocysteine levels in many people. Studies have shown that folic acid deficiency may be responsible for 15% to 20% of heart attacks and strokes in men (women have not yet been studied). Folic acid is involved in converting the amino acid homocysteine into another amino acid, methionine (by adding a single carbon, as a methyl group, to a sulfur atom). To a chemist, the term *homo* means that there is one additional carbon atom present. Homocysteine in the blood damages artery walls and causes heart attacks, but the mechanism by which homocysteine contributes to heart disease has not been fully identified. In 1997, the government's heart-health promoters continued to ignore the issue of homocysteine in favor of cholesterol, arguing that there was not yet sufficient evidence regarding the former. At that time, clinical analyses of homocysteine in blood were difficult to obtain, but these analyses are now available, and many physicians presently recognize high homocysteine levels as a hazard. In the future, blood may be checked routinely for homocysteine levels as it now is for cholesterol levels as an indicator of heart attack risk.

Our bodies produce homocysteine by removing a methyl group from the natural amino acid methionine, which is derived from protein in our diets. The B vitamins help an enzyme in the liver convert homocysteine back into methionine. When there is a deficiency of these vitamins, the higher levels of homocysteine ravage the blood vessels. These B vitamins occur in many foods but are very easily destroyed by processing. People who have high homocysteine levels in their blood may have aberrant forms of the gene controlling the transformation of homocysteine to methionine. Thus, part of this problem is genetic, but diet and supplements of folic acid and vitamins B_{12} and B_6 can help lower high homocysteine concentrations to safe levels (<14 micromoles per liter).

During their reproductive years, women's homocysteine levels are roughly 20% lower than men's, but after menopause, their homocysteine levels and heart-disease risk rise to match those of men. In old age, both sexes experience increased homocysteine levels as their bodies become less efficient at absorbing vitamin B_{12}.

Vitamin B_6 (pyridoxine) is essential to protein metabolism. B_6 is found in cereals, potatoes, milk, meat, and beer. The average daily intake of B_6 is about 2 mg, which is a little more than the sufficient body requirement. Many women take this vitamin to combat pre-menstrual syndrome. Some vitamin advocates have suggested taking up to 200 mg per day. A British health minister warns that prolonged high doses of B_6 are associated with peripheral neuropathy, a neurological disorder that leads to numbness and clumsiness in the hands and feet. To avoid this problem, take no more than 100 mg daily.

Fat-soluble vitamins dissolve in oily liquids rather than in water. One of them, vitamin K, is required for normal blood clotting. Vitamin A (retinol) is the precursor of a light-sensitive group of visual pigments. A deficiency of vitamin A results in night blindness; young animals also require retinol for growth. Although the vitamin is vital for good vision and a healthy immune system, when consumed in excess, vitamin A is toxic. This may be why Eskimos avoid eating polar bear livers, which are rich in this vitamin.

Vitamin D, the "sunshine vitamin," has an interesting history. This vitamin is normally manufactured in the skin by the action of sunlight, which converts a cholesterol derivative into vitamin D. Most foods have a very low, insufficient level of vitamin D. An exception is cod-liver oil, which was fed to children in cloudy England to prevent rickets, a disease characterized by inadequate calcium uptake in cartilage and bone. Rickets was once called the "children's disease of the English." Bedouin Arab women have a vitamin D deficiency because only their eyes are exposed to sunlight; they are thus subject to osteomalacia—weakening of the bones. In the western world, vitamin D is now added as a fortificant to milk (400 IU per quart). A 1998 study showed that even among young, healthy people taking vitamin D supplements, more than 40% were deficient in vitamin D. Part of this problem may stem from underexposure to sunlight. People in northern latitudes make almost no vitamin D in their skin in winter, so this group, as well as those who are home bound, are also vulnerable. Older people are advised to consume up to 600 IU of vitamin D a day; this recommendation may be raised to 800 IU despite potential toxicity of high doses.

In the liver and kidneys, vitamin D is converted to an active hormone, calcitrol, by the addition of hydroxyl (OH) groups. Calcitrol is essential to the control of calcium and phosphorus metabolism and for the adsorption of these nutrients. In old age, the enzymes that carry out this transformation may become impaired. Calcitrol may become available in the future as a drug.

Is "Health Food Store" an Oxymoron?

Vitamin E, alpha-tocopherol, has been much in the news. This vitamin is another antioxidant that is thought to take up reactive oxygen species, thereby protecting coronary arteries against atherosclerosis and DNA against attacks by these chemical carcinogens. Vitamin E may also prevent premature aging in normal cells throughout the body. People consuming low-fat diets can become deficient in vitamin E, and this deficiency may be exacerbated by vigorous exercise, resulting in toxic levels of reactive oxygen species. It is claimed that vitamin E reduces muscle soreness when taken before vigorous exercise.

Recent studies suggest that large doses of vitamin E may prevent heart disease and cancer. At high levels, vitamin E prevents oxidation of LDL cholesterol, the "bad" cholesterol—thus curbing the LDL's ability to latch on to artery walls and form the clogging plaque associated with coronary heart disease. To prevent heart disease, the combination of vitamin E with aspirin is thought to be more effective than aspirin alone. Earlier evidence that vitamin E is an anticancer agent was based only on animal studies; however, this evidence has now been buttressed by a Finnish study of adult men showing that vitamin E supplements reduced prostate cancer risk by one-third. Studies with senior patients have also shown that vitamin E supplements can improve immunologic responses. In 1996, researchers found that postmenopausal women who have the highest vitamin E intake from their food—up to 10 IU per day—are less likely to die of heart disease than those consuming less.

Some proponents claim that the levels of vitamin E necessary for these beneficial effects cannot be obtained through diet alone—40 times more may be needed as a supplement (a minimum dose of 400 IU). This level of supplementation should be considered a drug. There are possible deleterious side effect to such high levels: bleeding problems have occurred in some people as well as increased blood pressure! Furthermore, double-blind tests on large patient groups have not yet been performed, so beware! It is also possible that, as an antioxidant, vitamin E may promote the growth of cancer cells once a cancer has been established.

Olive oil is rich in a biologically effective form of vitamin E. Other sources are wheat germ, nuts, green leafy vegetables, beans, and avocados. These foods contain a second form, gamma vitamin E, which protects the body against nitrogen oxides either from polluted air or from inflammation produced by the body's immune system.

This gamma form is not found in most vitamin supplements; furthermore, high doses of the more common alpha form are claimed to deplete the body's reserves of the gamma form. These contradictory effects leave the average person in a quandary.

Hormone Supplements

Most people have heard the word *hormone,* but what is a hormone? This word is derived from the Greek word meaning "to spur on." Hormones are chemical messengers made in endocrine glands. They are secreted directly into the blood, which then carries them to their sites of action, where they alter the activities of responsive tissues. A single hormone molecule can have a very large effect, for example, by turning on an enzyme that itself produces many thousands of other molecules or events. There are many kinds of hormones, but in this section I will consider only hormones that you can purchase in health food stores, and environmental chemicals that simulate hormones.

The simplest hormone, nitric oxide (NO), is a potent vasodilator and can counteract the vasoconstrictive effect of nicotine, thus enhancing nicotine uptake from cigarettes. This hormone is also a known combustion product from ammonium and nitrate salts. The latter have been found in surprisingly high levels as additives in commercial cigarettes. Some scientists have proposed that these NO-forming dopants were added to enhance nicotine uptake from cigarette smoke, rather than to lower tobacco's acidity, as was claimed.

NO is made from a natural amino acid, arginine, by the enzyme NO synthase. A similar molecule, asymmetric dimethylarginine (ADMA) is a naturally occurring analog of arginine. As a structural cousin of arginine, ADMA inhibits the enzyme that produces NO in the body, thus lowering the concentration of NO. Elevated ADMA levels in a patient's blood have been correlated with the severity of vasodilator dysfunction. A high level of ADMA is considered a risk factor that may correlate with heart disease better than LDL, the "bad" cholesterol.

You might ask: because it occurs naturally in the body, how can one control high ADMA levels? One answer is to deliver supplemental arginine, which has a bitter taste. A nonprescription medical

Is "Health Food Store" an Oxymoron?

food in the form of a candy bar containing arginine has come on the market; it is available in some health food stores under the name HeartBar. Clinical studies show that eating two of these bars a day can reduce symptoms in patients with coronary heart disease. Each bar contains 3 grams of arginine. This medical candy should be used only after consultation with a physician. Because NO is also involved in inflammation, these arginine-rich candy bars should be avoided by patients with arthritis.

Melatonin

Melatonin is a natural hormone secreted by the pineal gland, a pea-size structure at the center of the brain, as shown in Figure 6. Melatonin is thought to reset the body's clock and to help sleep without the hazards or side effects of prescription sleeping pills. However, a double-blind Norwegian study of melatonin's effect on jet lag failed to show any effect!

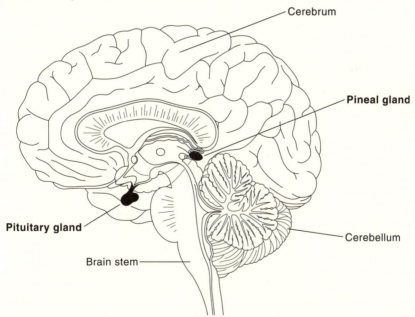

Figure 6. Pineal and pituitary glands are the sites in the brain where many hormones (such as melatonin and oxytocin) are secreted.

Is "Health Food Store" an Oxymoron?

There has been a melatonin frenzy the past few years. Until 1996, melatonin was available only in health food stores; now it can be purchased over the counter in conventional drugstores. The amount of melatonin taken by the public must be very large. Many commercial samples of melatonin are probably not synthesized under the carefully documented manufacturing protocols required by the FDA for traditional pharmaceuticals. Numerous claims have been made for melatonin beyond inducing sleep. Animal tests suggest that melatonin protects cells and slows the growth of tumors by strengthening the immune system. Incredible claims made for melatonin include that it can extend your life span to 120 years, reverse the aging process, and reinvigorate your sex life. For many, the lure of a safe, cheap, natural panacea is irresistible. In the absence of thorough studies, however, you would be wise to be skeptical. Upon closer inspection, many of the claims about the health benefits of melatonin turn out to be merely hypotheses with little supporting data.

What about the melatonin naturally produced in our bodies? The tiny pineal gland is a regulator; it controls the body's biological clock through excretion of melatonin, primarily at night when we sleep. In animals, the pineal gland is thought to have many other regulatory roles: sexual arousal, bird migration, and signaling of hibernation. Humans first obtain melatonin from breast milk when they are infants, and later their own pineal glands manufacture it. Melatonin levels rise through childhood, drop during adolescence, and then steadily decline with age. The steepest decline occurs from age 50 on. By age 60 we produce about half the melatonin we did at 20.

The smallest commercial dose of melatonin is 1 milligram (equivalent to about one grain of table salt). The usual recommended dose is 3 milligrams, and the highest dose recommended to induce sleep is 6 to 10 milligrams. Our bodies produce about 0.3 milligram per day, but remember that melatonin is synthesized in the brain, where it is active. An oral dose of melatonin must first pass through the stomach and then through the liver before it has the opportunity to cross from the blood via the blood–brain barrier into the brain, where it is thought to exert its biological action.

No drug or biomolecule is without side effects, and that is true of melatonin. Up to 10% of people taking melatonin have complained of nightmares, headaches, morning grogginess, mild depression, and low sex drive. Melatonin should be avoided by pregnant and nursing mothers (no one knows its effect on a fetus or infant), as well as by people with allergies or autoimmune diseases (perhaps including some diabetics), healthy children (who make enough of their own), and women trying to get pregnant. Melatonin can act as a contraceptive and has been studied in the Netherlands for that purpose.

Steroid hormones

Steroids contain four rings of carbon atoms; some steroids function as hormones in animals. The steroid hormones are made from cholesterol in various glands (liver, testes, ovaries, and adrenal) by enzymes that use molecular oxygen.

Steroid hormones are often in the news, especially the male sex hormone testosterone and the female sex hormone estrogen. Estrogen is a general term for female sex hormones such as estradiol and estrone. Testosterone and estrogen are responsible for male and female secondary sex characteristics, respectively. The male hormones, called androgens, promote the growth of facial hair and muscle in men.

Testosterone levels are clearly related to emotion. In both monkeys and humans, testosterone levels rise sharply in combat and victory and fall after defeat, either in physical battle or during mental games such as chess. There is also evidence that these fluctuations occur in onlookers! A study of testosterone in saliva samples from "rabid" soccer fans demonstrated this rise or fall of testosterone with victory or defeat, respectively.

The female sex hormone estrogen protects younger women against heart attacks and helps retain calcium, thereby reducing a woman's chance of developing osteoporosis. Estrogen is also thought to enhance memory and other mental functions. After menopause, a woman's estrogen level falls. Many postmenopausal women start hormone-replacement therapy (HRT), but others choose not to do so because of the associated increased risk of uterine and breast cancer. This "balancing act" leaves women with a difficult, personal choice between two hazards. Preliminary data from a large federal study indicate that initially, HRT may not protect postmenopausal women from heart disease and may even lead to a tiny increase in risk for heart attacks, strokes, and blood clots in the legs and lungs. These sorts of health claims should always be treated with caution; very large, rigorous, double-blind studies carried out over a long period are required to reach a final judgment in such matters.

Although testosterone is commonly known as a male sex hormone, women also produce testosterone in their ovaries (at about one-twentieth of male levels). After surgical removal of the uterus and ovaries, women require low doses of testosterone, which can be administered by injections, implants, or an experimental transdermal skin patch. Although steroid hormones are natural, most cannot be purchased without a doctor's prescription.

Football players at all levels in the United States as well as other athletes have taken anabolic steroids to enhance their athletic performance. Until recently, this dubious practice was limited primarily to males. A study in 1997 reported that as many as 175,000 high school girls in the United States have used steroids. They take these illegal drugs to become leaner and to build more muscle. The side effects are shocking: shrinkage of their breasts, male-hair growth, deepening of the voice, and menstrual problems. Like a tattoo, these effects can become permanent, but unlike a tattoo, they are serious health threats. Other long-term problems include cardiovascular, liver, and reproductive illnesses.

Dehydroepiandrosterone (DHEA) is a steroid hormone manufactured in the human adrenal gland. Because it is also considered a naturally occurring food supplement, DHEA supplements are not under the control of the FDA. As such, these supplements can be purchased in health food stores in the United States.

DHEA is termed a *precursor hormone* because it is subsequently converted into both estrogen and testosterone in the body. There is more DHEA circulating in a person than any other hormone, but the amount depends on age. DHEA is produced most abundantly in young adults and then declines as people age. By age 80, our DHEA levels are only 5% of the peak level reached by most people between ages 18 and 30. DHEA has been promoted as a "miracle antiaging" food supplement that could give a 50-year-old "couch potato" the sexual performance of a 20 year old! Is DHEA effective and safe? Hormones are not cough drops! Some hormones have powerful and multiple effects on human health. By 1999, at least 21 studies of DHEA had been done in people, but no clear answers have emerged. There is no clear-cut beneficial outcome of DHEA supplementation, but there are some troubling findings, particularly about its use in women. High, natural levels of DHEA in premenopausal women have been linked to a lower risk of breast cancer, but postmenopausal women who had the highest DHEA levels also had the highest risk of breast cancer. In women, DHEA supplements have been associated with side effects such as the growth of unwanted facial hair, baldness, a deepening voice, and acne. No other country with a regulatory system for drugs allows DHEA to be sold over the counter. In Canada, it cannot be obtained even by prescription. One may ask, then, why DHEA is sold over the counter in the United States, for it is neither a natural medicine nor a true dietary supplement.

Peptide hormones

Peptides (small proteins) can be hormones; one of the most celebrated examples is insulin, which controls the levels of glucose (a sugar) in the blood. High levels of insulin in the blood signal the body that it is well fed, and low levels indicate low blood sugar levels. Most readers have heard of the genetic disease diabetes, in which glucose is overproduced in the liver and is underutilized by other organs. Diabetes is the most common serious metabolic disease in the world; it affects millions. It got its name in the 2nd century A.D. because of the excessive urination associated with the disease. About 6% of the US population has one or another form of diabetes. Type 1 diabetes is the result of insufficient insulin production. Other types of diabetes are less well understood. Most diabetic patients must inject themselves with insulin and monitor their blood sugar levels several times a day. When there is too little insulin in the blood, excess glucose builds up, which over time can lead to serious side effects such as blindness and kidney damage. Too much insulin is also dangerous and may cause insulin shock. If the blood sugar level drops too low, hypoglycemia can result, which can also be life threatening. Insulin is available only by prescription. It is either isolated from pigs or manufactured using recombinant DNA techniques.

Other hormonal peptides can also be manufactured using recombinant DNA. Usually, hormonal peptides must be administered by injection, because enzymes in the stomach would digest orally administered peptides by breaking their amide bonds. One such hormonal peptide is the nonapeptide (literally, nine amino acids) called oxytocin. Oxytocin is produced in the pituitary gland and helps control the contraction of the uterus during childbirth. Sometimes this hormone is given to stimulate labor.

The peptide hormone erythropoietin (EPO) stimulates production of red blood cells, which carry oxygen throughout the body. This natural substance is produced by genetic-engineering techniques and is used as a drug for patients receiving kidney dialysis (EPO is made in the kidneys). Some athletes "dope" themselves with this hormone to improve their performance in endurance sports. Their pulse rates are about half those of most other people. Such blood doping is illegal, but the detection of additional quantities of this natural hormone is nearly impossible. This doping has a dangerous side effect, because EPO thickens the blood. Some bicycle racers are thought to have died from erythropoietin doping. The hormone is believed to cause heart attacks while the riders sleep. In 1998, a French racing team was banned from the famous month-long Tour de France race because their coach had allegedly provided them with EPO. This is an excellent illustration of an inappropriate use of a natural substance that can cause death, even in well-conditioned adults. Fortunately, this natural hormone is not available in health food stores, but there are illegal sources.

Somatotropin is another small protein hormone normally synthesized in the pituitary gland. A deficiency of this human growth hormone (HGH) produces dwarfism, and an excess leads to gigantism. In adults, levels of HGH taper off gradually after middle age. Dwarf children have been successfully treated with HGH isolated from the pituitary glands of cadavers, but in rare cases, HGH from this source is contaminated with a dangerous virus. The advent of genetic engineering has allowed the manufacture of larger quantities of HGH as well as the closely related bovine growth hormone (BGH). Synthetic HGH is now used to treat dwarfs, but there are three unauthorized black markets for this powerful peptide hormone: for short but not dwarf children, for geriatric individuals, and for body builders. Although it can legally be obtained by prescription, HGH can be purchased through the internet as well.

In the first unethical use, it is suspected that some normal children or teenagers are being given HGH to stimulate growth beyond their normal stature. The extent of this practice is unclear. The unethical use of HGH by body builders is not well documented or well studied. The use of HGH as a "fountain of youth" for seniors is illegal in the United States except in authorized clinical research. A landmark medical study, published in 1990, reported the results of injecting HGH three times a week into 12 men aged 61 to 81. After only 6 months of growth hormone injections, these subjects lost 14% of their body fat, gained nearly 9% in muscle mass, and had increased skin thickness and bone density comparable to levels typical of much younger adults. Anecdotal reports also indicated increased sexual vitality. Other beneficial effects attributed to HGH are more rapid healing and better sleep (more REM, rapid-eye-movement, sleep). Some older people taking HGH believe that you can't turn back the clock, but you can wind it up again! Antiaging clinics for both men and women have sprung up in Mexico, Switzerland, and in the United States, where patients can inject themselves with HGH for about $1,000 per month. The price is expected to fall.

Is HGH really a fountain of youth? Does it arrest aging for those who can afford it? Perhaps not—and there are serious side effects. Crippling cases of carpal tunnel syndrome have been reported. These cases appear related to the hormone's overstimulation of cartilage growth in the wrists, resulting in inflammation of neighboring nerves. Diabetes-like symptoms and enlarged, tender breasts in males have also been reported. These adverse side effects may be related to the dose level, which may need to be adjusted according to the individual. More must be learned about this supposed antiaging drug before it can be considered safe to use.

There is a fourth use of growth hormone. You may have read about BGH. BGH is manufactured by recombinant DNA techniques and injected into dairy cows to increase milk production, reportedly by up to 25%. Environmental groups and dairy farmers have fought over the introduction and use of BGH. Some groups have attempted to require labeling of milk products produced with BGH supplements. All cows have natural levels of BGH, traces of which appear in the milk. As a protein, BGH is degraded into amino acids when the milk is metabolized in your stomach. It is nearly impossible to detect BGH supplements in milk. Many scientists believe that milk from BGH-treated cows should have no effect on anyone who drinks such milk.

Performance-Enhancing Drugs

Performance-enhancing drugs have been used by athletes as far back as 500 B.C., when opiates were taken to improve performance. Some of these natural substances enhance performance, but they may be dangerous. You have already learned about the misuse of some steroid hormones and of EPO.

You may have heard about a new product in the health food stores, HMb. This substance is a natural metabolite, and as such, HMb can be manufactured and sold without control by the FDA— provided that it is not advertised as a medicine. What is HMb? It is the calcium salt of beta-hydroxy, beta-methylbutyric acid. HMb is thought to minimize protein breakdown and damage to muscles.

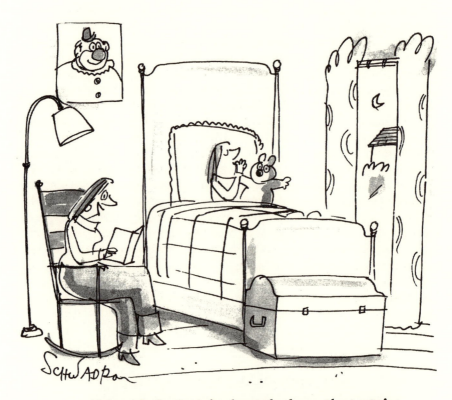

"Although the tortoise beat the hare, the tortoise was later disqualified for taking anabolic steroids, so the hare was declared the winner."

Is "Health Food Store" an Oxymoron?

Livestock-feeding studies suggest this additive increases the protein to fat ratio. More significant is a reported study on Iowa State football players suggesting that HMb helps retain muscle protein after strenuous exercise. Here is a legal, apparently performance-enhancing drug! Amateur body builders and people interested in maximizing their muscle mass have become interested in HMb as information about it is passed by word of mouth or by stories in trade magazines. The suggested dose of this additive is four 250-mg pills (1 gram), three times a day! A bottle containing 120 pills (a 10-day supply) was priced in the year 2000 at $34.95. The side effects, if any, are not clear, but any such effects may be slowly discovered and reported anecdotally. Thus, its safety remains in question.

Another controversial performance-enhancing chemical is andro stenedione, dubbed "andro." This steroid is the precursor of the male sex hormone testosterone. Andro was thought to raise levels of testosterone, thus building lean muscle and promoting recovery from injury. Over the long term, such anabolic steroids can cause fatal side effects including heart attacks, cancer, liver dysfunction, severe mood disorders, and mental dysfunction. Andro was the performance enhancer of choice by the East German sports machine, whose athletes used it through the 1988 Olympics in Seoul, Korea. After that time, the development of a method for detecting andro led to its demise.

The FDA has classified andro as a dietary supplement; therefore, it can be purchased in health food stores. Even though its use had already been banned by the National Football League, National Collegiate Athletic Association, and the Olympics, andro was still permitted in professional baseball as of the year 2000. In 1998, andro became controversial after home-run hitter Mark McGwire of the St. Louis Cardinals admitted using this potentially dangerous steroid. Because of the publicity given McGwire's 70-homer season, sales of andro in the United States rose to $100 million per year. Then in 1999, a surprising study of males showed that andro may have increased the size of McGwire's breasts but not his muscles! Andro supplements taken by men raised their levels of the female hormone estrogen, but not those of testosterone. No increase in muscle development was detected in this test group. This finding is in contrast to a 1962 study that showed that andro does raise testosterone levels in women. This is an interesting example of differences that can occur in the metabolism of males and females. A later study, in February, 2000, showed that larger doses of andro, 300 milligrams per day, did increase testosterone levels in men.

THE FAR SIDE

By GARY LARSON

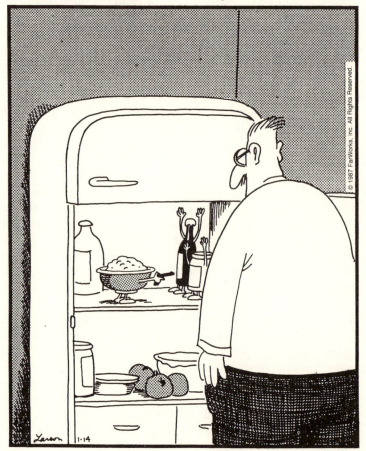

When potato salad goes bad

CHAPTER

4

Infectious Agents:
Are All Microorganisms Bad?

HUMAN DISEASES are often caused by microorganisms, such as bacteria, viruses, or fungi. Most people have heard about these naturally occurring microbes, but few understand what distinguishes a virus from a bacterium or whether all microorganisms are dangerous. It is important to realize that these organisms can multiply, either because they are alive or because they can command a cell to reproduce copies of themselves. Because of their ability to reproduce over a relatively short period of time, even a small number of microorganisms can lead to a serious infection. Microbes have another important characteristic. Because these organisms can change through modification of their DNA—a process referred to as mutation—or by exchange of genetic material with other microbes, initially benign microorganisms may become hazardous. Just as we found with chemicals, however, not all microorganisms are dangerous. In fact, some microorganisms are useful and even necessary for our well being.

Viruses

A virus is either one of the most complicated nonliving substances or one of the simplest living things we know about, depending on how we define "living." A virus consists of the genetic substances DNA or RNA encased in a distinctive protein coat. RNA viruses are called retroviruses. The protein coat protects the DNA or RNA and acts like a hypodermic needle to inject the DNA or RNA into a host cell. During this process, the virus sheds its protein overcoat.

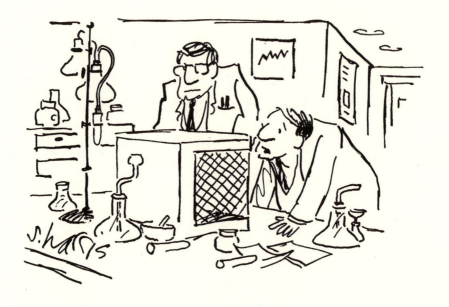

"BIGGEST DAMN VIRUS I'VE EVER SEEN!"

Viruses reproduce by infecting specific cells in an organism. Once a virus has entered the host cell, the viral DNA inserts itself into the cell's genetic databank and instructs the cell to make copies of the infecting virus, including its distinctive protein coat. You could describe this invasion as a genetic overthrow of the host cell. Virus production can take place to such an extent that the host cell will burst and die. This is the usual way that viruses kill cells and at the same time multiply.

Because they are incapable of independent growth, viruses are not really alive. In principle, a virus could last for a thousand years. Because it does not eat, a virus does not need to be fed. The virus's lifestyle explains why viral diseases are difficult to treat. Antibiotics are ineffective against viral infections. On the other hand, a virus can

Table 4   Viral infections and their modes of transmission[a]

Infectious disease	Infectious agent	Mode of transmission
AIDS virus infection	Human immuno-deficiency virus (HIV)	Sexual contact; sharing hypodermic needles; mother to child; blood product infusion before March 1985
Chickenpox*	Varicella-zoster virus (herpes zoster virus)	Airborne droplets; direct contact
Common cold	Numerous rhinoviruses; coronaviruses	Airborne droplets; hand-to-hand contact
Hepatitis, viral*	Hepatitis virus types A and B; others	Infected food or water (type A); sexual contact; blood-borne transmission; sharing hypodermic needles (type B)
Influenza*	Influenza viruses types A, B, or C	Airborne droplets
Measles*	Measles virus (a paramyxovirus)	Airborne droplets
Meningitis, viral	Various viruses	Various methods, including via rodents
Mononucleosis, infectious	Epstein-Barr virus	Possibly via saliva
Rabies*	Rabies virus (a rhabdovirus)	Bite from infected animal
Rubella*	Rubella virus	Airborne droplets; mother to child

[a]From Clayman, C. B., ed. 1989. *Encyclopedia of medicine.* The American Medical Association, New York: Random House, p. 584.

Asterisk (*) indicates disease for which a vaccine exists.

be destroyed by radiation. The best defense we have against viruses is vaccination, a process that mobilizes the body's immune system to attack a particular virus. Some important infectious viruses and their modes of transmission to humans are listed in Table 4.

Viruses have two weaknesses and at least one strength that are important in understanding viral diseases. The first weakness arises because viruses can bind and enter only specific kinds of cells. For this reason, viruses are usually species-specific. Viruses that infect cows do not easily infect humans, and when they do, the resulting disease is often attenuated. There are important exceptions to this rule. For example, the rabies virus can infect most mammalian species equally. In fact, you could get rabies from eating meat from a rabid animal, but this type of transmission is very rare because rabid animals do not get to the slaughterhouse! The second weakness of viruses is that irradiation of viruses with gamma rays causes mutations and breaks in their DNA and RNA molecules. Unlike whole cells, such as bacteria and muscle cells, viruses have no independent means of DNA or RNA repair. So, ionizing radiation can more easily "kill" a virus than it can a bacterium.

A major strength of viruses is their ability to mutate more readily than bacteria do. These mutations can change the protein coat on the virus, which is the part of the virus that the immune system recognizes in selecting a viral particle for destruction. A mutated virus may not be attacked by an immune defense previously developed to resist the virus's ancestors. Retroviruses, which contain fragile single strands of RNA, are more susceptible to mutations than viruses containing the more robust double-stranded DNA. For example, acquired immune-deficiency syndrome (AIDS) is caused by a retrovirus that readily undergoes mutations, altering its protein coat. This facile mutation is one reason that AIDS is difficult to resist. The human immunodeficiency virus (HIV) that causes AIDS is quick to develop resistance to antiviral drugs because of its rapid mutation rate, far faster than that of viruses of the common cold and other viruses. The new generation of AIDS viruses may not look anything like the prior form. A drug may kill most of the viral offspring, but the progeny with drug-resistant mutations survive. In Darwinian fashion, survival of the fittest, this mutation produces a new generation of super-resilient virus. A more effective treatment for AIDS is to confront the virus simultaneously with several drugs, each of which interferes with the virus's replication in the hope that it is forced to stop reproducing. A virus that cannot multiply cannot mutate. It is because of their rapid mutation that very few vaccines are effective against retroviruses. Another reason that AIDS is such a deadly disease is that the AIDS virus attacks and disarms the immune system, which is the body's last line of defense against all virus infections.

Viruses cause a large variety of human diseases and much suffering. The common cold and influenza are caused by viruses. Lest you think these are fairly minor ailments, consider the influenza epidemic of 1918. Estimates are that 21 million people died worldwide, more than were killed in World War I. The last influenza pandemic killed about 100,000 people in the United States alone. If it were unleashed throughout the world, the Ebola virus would probably cause a lethal pandemic.

Some viruses can be transferred between swine and humans; in this way, new epidemics of human influenza often have their origins in swine viruses. Virtually all influenza viruses originate in Asia, where the close proximity of humans with domestic swine, ducks, and chickens allows these microorganisms to swap genetic material, resulting in new viral strains. Typically, viruses pass from poultry to pigs and then to humans. Antibodies taken from survivors of the 1918 pandemic have been traced to a swine virus. The fact that viruses native to pigs are able to infect human cells raises concerns about cross-species organ transplants. For example, pig valves are commonly transplanted into human hearts.

Any influenza virus that can pass directly from poultry to humans, such as one reported from Hong Kong in 1997, can be particularly virulent. Since most influenza viruses come from pigs they are similar to previous influenza strains for which humans have developed antibodies. In contrast, because an avarian virus is so different, these antibodies would be completely ineffective against it. Thus, humans would be very susceptible to this pathogen, especially if it can be transferred between people and thus spread though the population. Carried by people traveling on airplanes, influenza viruses are almost unique in their ability to spread rapidly throughout the world. Travel around the world can be accomplished in less than 80 hours (compared with the 80 days of Jules Verne's 19th-century fantasy). In the 21st century, more than a million passengers, each a potential carrier of pathogens, travel daily by aircraft to international designations. With today's transportation system, a new virus for which we have no immunity could spread to every continent on Earth before disease-control centers even know it exists. You can understand why viruses pose a serious threat to humanity. The spread of hypervirulent viruses such as Ebola from Africa or the hantavirus from the US Southwest could threaten the general public, but so far, they have not.

Numerous other viral diseases are spread through food, typically by the fecal-oral route. This transmission occurs when someone does not wash their hands before serving or preparing food, thus contaminating the food and spreading the virus to anyone who eats this food. In this way, an outbreak of the viral disease hepatitis A can be caused by a single worker in a fast-food restaurant. You can understand that the viral infection was not inherent in the food itself. The food is merely the medium for transmitting the virus from one human to another, where it can enter the host's cells and multiply. For this reason, viral diseases are not effectively controlled by irradiation of food. Ordinarily, food doesn't carry viruses.

Monkeypox, a close relative of smallpox that causes a nearly indistinguishable disease, was reported in the 1990s in the Democratic Republic of Congo. These cases appear to be transmitted from human to human. Human smallpox was thought to have been eradicated. For this reason, smallpox vaccine has not been used in nearly two decades, leaving a population that could be vulnerable to monkeypox.

Type I diabetes, the variety that appears in young people, has long been considered to be inherited. This is an autoimmune disorder in which the body's immune system destroys the insulin-producing cells in the pancreas. Evidence now suggests that type I diabetes may have originated from a retrovirus that infected some ancestor long ago and incorporated its genes into the human genome. The clue comes from remnants of a protein once used to construct the outer surface of this ancient virus. Patients with this disease show genes from this retrovirus, but people without the disease show no evidence for this viral gene. This is an interesting example showing that genetic information can be introduced into higher organisms from a virus.

Not all viruses are dangerous; some are potentially useful antibiotics. For example, bacteriophages, which are among the most common organisms on Earth, are viral predators that attack bacteria. These tiny phages, approximately one-fortieth the size of a bacterium, kill bacteria with chilling efficiency. They latch onto the walls of bacterial cells and, like living syringes, inject their genetic material into the cells, taking over the bacteria's genetic machinery and directing the bacterium to make copies of the phage. As the phages multiply inside the bacterium, the bacterium's cell walls rupture, spilling out multiple copies of the phage. As is typical of other viruses, bacteriophages are very selective, attacking only one variety of bacteria. Bacteriophages have been developed as therapeutic agents, principally in the former Soviet Union. These agents are being studied in the United States as an alternative treatment for antibiotic-resistant bacteria such as the deadly *Staphylococcus aureus*. There are advantages to bacteriophages as therapeutic agents: they do not need to be fed, and they multiply as they are being used. However, they also have disadvantages: they must be refrigerated until used, and the immune system may attack them as foreign bodies. Furthermore, their debris may be toxic to the human host. Bacteriophages are presently widely employed as drugs in Georgia (a former Soviet republic); in the future, they may be used in the western world to replace antibiotics in the treatment of particular infections.

Bacteria

There are many types of bacteria; some are innocuous, whereas others are lethal. Examples of bacteria that cause important infectious diseases, along with their modes of transmission and methods of treatment, are listed in Table 5. Bacteria are primitive organisms re-

Table 5   Bacterial infections, their modes of transmission, and their treatment[a]

Infectious disease	Infectious agent	Mode of transmission	Treatment
Gonorrhea	*Neisseria gonorrhea*	Sexual contact; mother to baby	Penicillin; ampicillin; other antibiotics for resistant forms
Meningitis,* bacterial	*Neisseria meningitides* (meningococcus); *Streptococcus pneumonia;* others	Mother to baby via vagina; infection reaching bloodstream from another organ	Antibiotic treatment
Pertussis* (whooping cough)	*Bordetella pertussis*	Airborne droplets	Erythromycin in early stage; small children may require hospitalization
Pneumonia	*Streptococcus pneumonia; Legionella pneumophila;* others	Airborne droplets	Antibiotics
Tuberculosis	*Mycobacterium tuberculosis*	Airborne transmission; cow's milk	Various antibiotics; possibly surgery
Typhoid fever*	*Salmonella typhus*	Food and water contaminated with infected feces	Several effective drugs, but fever takes a long time to control

[a]From Clayman, C. B., ed. 1989. *Encyclopedia of medicine.* The American Medical Association, New York: Random House, p. 585.

Asterisk (*) indicates disease for which a vaccine is available.

ferred to as prokaryotes. In contrast to higher organisms, bacterial cells have no nucleus (a membrane-bound structure that contains the DNA). Rather, the DNA in bacteria floats about inside the cell, usually as a circle with no beginning or end. Bacterial cells are surrounded by a membrane made of lipid bilayers, and this membrane is encased by a sturdy carbohydrate capsule. This cell wall is the focus of attack on bacteria. Antibiotics such as penicillin destroy certain bacteria by interfering with the construction of their cell walls. Bacteria can survive and reproduce as long as they have food and the proper medium. Some bacteria can reproduce very rapidly—a single cell could divide into one billion cells in eight hours!

Bacteria can either be friend or foe, depending on the setting. For example, *Escherichia coli* (*E. coli*) bacteria found in the human digestive system are responsible for helping digest the material exiting the stomach, and they help keep out other bacteria that might cause disease. This is why taking a broad-spectrum antibiotic that kills our normal intestinal bacteria can result in an upset stomach. Temporary destruction of our "home-team" microbes provides an entry for "unfriendly" competitors. Representative, "good" bacteria—species such as *Lactobacillus* and *Bifidobacteria*—are familiar ingredients in live yogurts. These "friendly" bacteria inhibit the growth of harmful bacteria such as *Salmonella* and *Listeria* in the gut. Live cultures containing these friendly bacteria have been shown to protect children against diarrhea diseases.

Your mouth is a year-round tropical paradise for friendly bacteria. Between 200 and 500 species are estimated to live in this balmy environment that provides constant moisture and a steady influx of nutrients. Most oral bacteria are not harmful, an exception being *Streptococcus mutans,* which digests sugar and gives off lactic acid. This bacterium is the principal cause of tooth decay. Your immune system does not attack your own oral bacteria for reasons that are uncertain, but it may attack another strain introduced from contact with another person. DNA fingerprinting of saliva samples shows that certain oral bacteria are inherited from one's mother, never from contact with the father; probably one route is through antibodies passed from mother to child during nursing. It is also interesting that some bacteria, such as *S. mutans,* are not passed between kissing couples, but a different bacterium, implicated in gum disease, may be passed and will survive the transmission.

Infectious Agents: Are All Microorganisms Bad?

Beneficial bacteria present in range chickens are far less prevalent in factory-farmed chickens, which often are infected with *Salmonella,* a leading cause of food-borne illness. About 20% of chickens are infected with *Salmonella.* Each year in the United States, there are between 800,000 and 4 million cases of human *Salmonella* infections, resulting in 960 to 1,960 deaths. In 1998, a new technique was approved to reduce *Salmonella* infections in factory-raised chickens by exposing them to Preempt, a mixture of 29 beneficial bacteria that occur naturally in chickens and are passed from mother hen to chick. In factory farming, the breeder hens do not stay with their chicks, so the treatment with Preempt provides the substitute bacterial exposure. This is an excellent example of the protection friendly bacteria offer toward infectious microorganisms.

In humans, there is a downside to useful gut bacteria: flatulence. These bacteria break down hard-to-digest carbohydrates by a process known as fermentation, thus producing odorless gases—hydrogen, carbon dioxide, and methane—and some foul-smelling sulfur compounds, such as hydrogen sulfide. These are excreted through the rectum. One might say "a bit of wind is a small price to pay for a happy gut." Flatus gas is passed about 14 times a day in healthy people, with a volume of between 25 and 100 milliliters on each occasion.

If a foreign *E. coli* strain is introduced into the digestive tract, the result may be nausea and diarrhea. Unfriendly bacteria use the host's nutrients to grow and reproduce, and they produce molecules toxic to their host.

The presence of certain bacteria in a wound is bad news for the afflicted. *Clostridium perfringens,* a bacterium found in soil, digests wounded flesh voraciously in a disease known as gangrene. This disease probably caused more deaths in the Civil War than did direct hits. The rifle bullets of the day were subsonic, which meant they did not get very hot in transit from the gun to the target. Thus, any organisms adhering to the bullet were carried alive into the wound. Worse yet, to make them easier to ram into the gun barrel, bullets were greased with lard, which provided a very hospitable environment for bacterial growth. This situation contributed to death tolls close to 50% in certain battles during the Civil War. In today's warfare, a death toll of 10% is viewed as a virtual bloodbath.

An organism that is presently not harmful to its host may not always remain so benign. How can such a transformation take place?

Every organism is defined by its DNA. An organism's genetic code is constantly being mutated by reactive oxygen species, ionizing radiation from the sun, and chemicals in the environment. Cellular machinery exists to correct this process, but it isn't 100% effective, so some mutations survive and are passed on to future generations. Most of the time, these mutations prove fatal, but occasionally one occurs that changes the cell's machinery in a favorable manner for the organism. An organism possessing such a favorable mutation is at an advantage for a particular niche, and consequently offspring are produced that have an easier life than their same-species competition. Bacteria can also exchange genes and thus transfer antibiotic resistance to their neighbors. Over time, mutations and gene transfers will result in an increased population of bacteria that have an advantageous trait. The ability of an organism to adapt like this is a good thing, because otherwise an environmental change could spell disaster for a particular species. However, a mutation benefiting a microorganism may make it dangerous to a host with which it is in contact.

An example of a transformation from a harmless to a deadly organism is the bacterium *Serratia marcescens.* Before the 1940s, this innocuous microbe was used as a valuable research tool. Oral surgeons exposed patients' gums to it during surgery. Subsequent blood tests demonstrated the possibility of blood infection by contamination from the oral cavity. In the 1950s and 1960s, the United States government spread this benign bacterium around the San Francisco Bay Area from aircraft to create a seemingly harmless scenario to study germ warfare. Over time, *Serratia* passed through many human immune systems and mutated, creating a species most dangerous to humans. This virulent form is now resistant to all but the most powerful antibiotics. In the early 1980s, workers in the Intensive Care Unit at Stanford University Hospital began seeing numerous patients experiencing symptoms of shock from blood infections caused by this bacteria. The US government's role in military research with this organism resulted in a wrongful death lawsuit that went all the way to the Supreme Court, where it was refused a hearing.

Bacterial agents are important in biological warfare. The most publicized example is anthrax, a disease caused by a bacterium, *Bacillus anthracis.* This bacterium produces spores that can survive dormant for many years in soils or animal products but are capable of reactivation. Animals can become infected by grazing on contaminated land, and people may be infected by contact with animals that have died of anthrax, by inhaling spores, or by eating infected meat. Anthrax is curable in its early stages with penicillin, but without immediate treatment, those who are exposed may die. In the United States, human cases are extremely rare, but the Soviets are known to have prepared biological bombs with anthrax spores, and the Iraqi regime under Saddam Hussein was discovered to be working on anthrax for biological warfare. Anthrax spores are easily transported and dispersed; thus, this agent is perhaps more dangerous than atomic weapons. Moreover, the dispersion of anthrax would not require a strong military power. A small plane, even an unmanned drone flying over Washington, DC, could disperse enough anthrax to kill several million people. Some American military force personnel have been vaccinated against this deadly bacterium, but the Soviets are known to have been preparing anthrax mutants that might be resistant to these vaccines.

Another biological warfare agent is now being used as a medicine and for cosmetic purposes! A highly dilute form of botulinum toxin (BTX), the deadly toxin that causes botulism, is being used by dermatologists to treat wrinkles! Even though this is a "natural" substance, if inhaled or ingested, a millionth of a gram of BTX can paralyze the lungs and cause asphyxiation. A billionth of a gram (one thousand-fold less) of BTX, injected in the forehead or in crow's feet, deactivates the nerves that normally command the muscles to contract, creating wrinkles. After treatment with "Botox," the skin flattens out, but the affected area must be reinjected after three or four months. As the first bacterial toxin to be approved by the FDA, Botox underwent one of the strictest approval trials ever conducted by the FDA. In fact, this therapeutic toxin was approved, not to remove wrinkles, but to treat involuntary muscle contraction. However, the law does not prevent doctors from using an approved drug for other purposes, and so Botox can be and is presently used legally for cosmetic purposes. A typical cosmetic treatment costs between $400 and $1,200 every four months. Sales are expected to reach $100 million per year. Who uses this stuff? Few admit to it. Patients have been said to line up in a waiting room "like sardines in sunglasses." It is amusing that research on deadly botulinum toxin would one day keep wealthy patients free from wrinkles! Botox should not be used by pregnant women.

Fungi

Fungi are a type of microorganism related to molds and yeasts. In some ways, fungi resemble tiny plants, but there are major differences. The cell walls of fungi are not made from cellulose, like plant cell walls are. Instead, cell walls in fungi are constructed of chitin, the carbohydrate-amine polymer that makes up the tough outer skeletons of lobsters and insects. Scientists refer to fungi as eukaryotic microorganisms, a higher life form than bacteria.

Many fungi such as mushrooms, morels, and truffles are edible. These foods are nutritional and delicious. On the other hand, most people know that certain similar-looking, wild mushrooms can be deadly! These naturally occurring, wild mushrooms are said to taste good, but they produce very toxic chemicals that can destroy your liver. Sometimes the only treatment for mushroom poisoning is a liver transplant! An unusual wild mushroom is the poisonous jack o'lantern *(Omphalotus olearius)* that masquerades by day as a member of the edible chanterelle family. By night, the jack o'lantern mushroom glows an "evil" yellow-green sufficiently bright to read a newspaper by.

By this point you have learned that most microbes are not intrinsically good or bad. Of paramount importance however, is *where* the microbe abides. In the wrong place, even useful microorganisms become harmful. For example, people who bake bread and fail to wash their hands afterward are at potential risk for a yeast infection from the baker's yeast *Saccheromyces cerevisiae.* The infection can cause a very unpleasant disease called thrush, which invades the oral cavity or vaginal tract of the victim. Fungi cause a variety of other human ailments. These include athlete's foot, ringworm, and respiratory problems.

Algae

You may have noticed green scum on the surface of a quiet pond. This is the result of microorganisms called algae, which are actually little plants. Sometimes algae are annoying to swimmers. The growth of algae also chokes oxygen out of the water so that fish have difficulty breathing. However, most common algae are not toxic, as evidenced by the sale of dry algae as a health food product. In certain circumstances, however, these single-cell aquatic organisms produce potent toxins that can kill people, cows, birds, and fish. For example, one type of dangerous algae is a dinoflagellate called *Pfiesteria,* a tiny creature covered with a cellulose armor plate. This aquatic organism produces several natural but toxic substances. One of its toxic products kills fish, and another opens up the fish's skin, allowing *Pfiesteria* to feed on the tissue inside.

In high concentrations, these dangerous algae form red or green tides. The microorganisms that cause red tides are called gymnodinium. Their red pigments are used for photosynthesis, like green chlorophyll in plants. Some of the oil deposits in the North Sea and elsewhere are the remains of ancient algae blooms that settled and accumulated on the ocean floor.

Toxic algae were apparently known in biblical times. The description in Exodus of a plague that turned the water blood-red and destroyed fish was probably a red tide. Mussels and other shellfish that feed on such microorganisms can accumulate the algal toxic byproducts with no apparent effect. When people eat shellfish harvested during a toxic tide, however, the results can be unpleasant and sometimes lethal. These colorless toxins are not destroyed by cooking and can produce gastrointestinal effects, dizziness, confusion, memory loss, or paralysis. Perhaps the prohibition against eating shellfish among Jews and Muslims stemmed from such events. Beachcombers can be exposed to airborne toxins from red tides, resulting in stinging sensations in their noses and throats. Some of these toxins are enzyme inhibitors, which act by locking onto and shutting down essential enzymes. Other toxins block nerve-cell channels, resulting in paralysis.

In recent years, there has been an increase in both the frequency and extent of harmful algal blooms in coastal waters that occur in many parts of the world. It has been proposed that this increased growth is the result of phosphorus and nitrogen nutrients washing off the land from sewage disposal and agricultural fertilizers. Increased traffic on the world's oceans may be a factor in spreading new blooms to previously algae-free water.

Lesser-Known Microorganisms

There are other types of microorganisms that also cause disease in humans. These organisms are neither bacteria or viruses. A few important examples are listed in Table 6, along with their modes of transmission and treatments. These pathological organisms can sometimes be treated with antibiotics that act by interfering with their life cycles.

Table 6   Other dangerous microorganisms, their modes of transmission, and their treatment[a]

Infectious disease	Infectious agent	Mode of transmission	Treatment
Nonspecific urethritis	*Chlamydia trachomatis*	Sexual contact	Antibiotics
Psittacosis	*Chlamydia psittaci*	Inhalation of dust containing feces from infected birds	Antibiotics
Q fever	*Coxiella burnetti*	Inhalation of infected dust	Antibiotics
Rocky Mountain spotted fever	*Rickettsia rickettsii*	Bite from infected tick	Antibiotics
Amebiasis	*Entamoeba histolytica*	Food and water contaminated by feces	Antiprotozoal drugs (e.g., metronidazole)
Giardiasis	*Giardia lamblia*	Food and water contaminated by feces; sexual contact	Antiprotozoal drugs (e.g., metronidazole)
Malaria	*Plasmodium falciparum; Plasmodium vivax;* others	Bite from infected mosquito	Various drugs (e.g., chloroquine)

[a]From Clayman, C. B., ed. 1989. *Encyclopedia of medicine.* The American Medical Association, New York: Random House, p. 586.

Infectious Agents: Are All Microorganisms Bad?

Chlamydiae are such a group of microorganisms. They are intermediate in size between bacteria and viruses and cause infectious
diseases in humans and animals (particularly birds). Like viruses,
they can multiply only by first invading the cells of another life form;
otherwise, they behave more like bacteria than viruses and are susceptible to treatment with antibiotic drugs.

Protozoa are microscopic, single-celled organisms larger than
bacteria. About 30 different types of protozoa are troublesome parasites of humans. Included are organisms that cause giardiasis (intestinal infections that result in diarrhea); and the insect-borne tropical
diseases malaria and sleeping sickness. With the advent of widespread air travel, giardia has spread across all parts of the United
States, so that it is no longer safe to drink from a clear spring or
stream even in the wildest parts of the mountains or forests. To be
safe, the water must be purified with chemicals such as iodine or fil-
tered through a micropore filter. The giardia organisms are transported about the wilderness by wild animals and are spread in the
animals' feces.

Rickettsiae are another type of parasitic microorganism. They
also resemble small bacteria, but are able to multiply only by invading the cells of another life form because they cannot produce their
own energy molecule, adenosine triphosphate (ATP). In this respect
they are more like viruses. Rickettsiae are primarily parasites of the
arthropods (insects and insectlike animals), such as lice, fleas, ticks,
and mites. These arthropods, however, can transmit rickettsiae to
larger animals (such as rodents, dogs, or humans) via the saliva of bit-
ing ticks or by depositing their feces on the skin, after which the
rickettsiae pass to the blood via a small skin break. Human diseases
caused by different types of rickettsiae include Rocky Mountain spot-
ted fever, Q fever, and various forms of typhus.

An insidious parasite, *Trypanosoma cruzi,* the vector (disease-
causing agent) of Chagas' disease, is carried by *R. prolixua,* a member
of the "kissing bug" family. While the insect is feeding, this parasite
is passed through the bug's feces into the victim's bloodstream. Once
there, the parasite usually infects and degrades heart muscle. The
presently incurable Chagas' disease is endemic to Central and South
America, where it is a serious public health problem. Between 16
and 18 million Latin Americans are presently infected with *T. cruzi;*
about 43,000 die annually of Chagas' disease. DNA analysis of mum-
mies from the Atacama desert on the west coast of South America in-

dicates that Chagas' disease infected and killed New World peoples as far back as 3000 B.C.

Few Americans are aware of Chagas' disease and the danger from the kissing bug. They should be! This disease and the kissing bug are present in the United States, mostly in Texas and Arizona. Approximately 300,000 people, most commonly migrants from Latin America, are thought to be infected. It is disturbing that Chagas' disease can be transmitted by blood transfusion and that blood donations in the United States are not yet being screened for this disease, even though precautionary analysis of donated blood is commonly employed in South America!

Mad-Cow and Related Prion Diseases

Whereas viruses, fungi, and bacteria are fairly well understood disease-causing agents, some mysterious diseases are caused by pathogens of less-certain origin. A vivid example is mad-cow disease, which decimated Britain's beef industry in 1992. The cause of this disease is controversial. There are a number of similar diseases, referred to as spongiform encephalopathies, that affect sheep, cattle, mink, deer, cats, elephants, mice, goats, monkeys, and humans. The spongiform encephalopathies are fatal, untreatable diseases for which there is no adequate method of diagnosis before death. They are characterized by the appearance of holes or spongelike deterioration in the brain tissue that can be detected postmortem. Some of these diseases can be passed from one species to another through ingestion or injection of diseased tissue—usually brain tissue. Mad-cow disease is thought to have been transferred to cattle by feeding them bone parts from infected sheep. A related disease, scrapie, has long been recognized in sheep, but has not been reported to affect humans.

A related brain disease in humans is kuru, which appears to be transmitted by the ingestion of brain (by head hunters), as is Creutz-feldt–Jacob disease, first described in 1920. These diseases cause slow mental degeneration of the victim. Eating squirrel brains, which is a strange custom in parts of rural Kentucky, may also transmit a fatal variant of mad-cow disease to humans.

Because of a large body of circumstantial evidence, many researchers now believe that rogue proteins called prions (pronounced

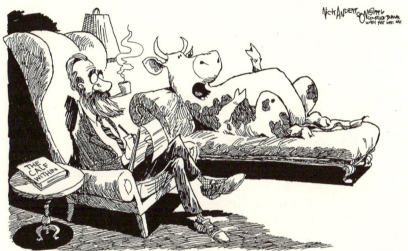

THE BRITISH GOVERNMENT ADDRESSES MAD-COW DISEASE

PREE-ons) are the villains behind mad-cow disease in cattle, Creutzfeldt–Jacob disease in humans, and all other spongiform encephalopathies. The term *prion* stands for "proteinaceous infectious particles." Strong evidence indicates that when tissue samples from the brains of people who died of Creutzfeldt–Jacob disease are injected into test animals, these animals develop a similar pattern of brain damage. The prion hypothesis states that the infectious agent is a renegade protein that can infect cells and make copies of itself. This mode of infection would require a unique mechanism of reproduction not involving DNA. A fundamental premise of biology is that DNA begets RNA, which begets protein. For the prion diseases, a new method of replication is proposed that involves an interaction between an abnormal prion protein and naturally occurring, non-pathogenic prion proteins normally found in animals. Proteins exist as helical coils and sheets that fold into the particular shapes necessary for their proper biological functions. The rogue prion protein is thought to have a different, sheetlike shape, and is thought to cause the normal ribbonlike, helical prion protein to change over to the more stable, sheetlike structure, thus forming insoluble plaques in the brain. This transformation would not require the production of many new protein molecules, but one proposal suggests that this physical transformation of the natural protein is initiated by a small number of abnormal proteins (Figure 7, see color section).

In 1997, the Nobel prize in Physiology or Medicine was awarded to Stanley B. Prusiner for the prion hypothesis. Nevertheless, some scientists still consider Prusiner's theory unproved. The evidence that a pure protein can cause the prion diseases is still not perfect. This theory does not easily explain the observation of long incubation times, which may last several years in humans. Another difficulty is that the infectious agent must pass through the digestive enzymes in the stomach and then penetrate the formidable blood–brain barrier. Doubts will remain about the prion hypothesis until someone injects a purified prion protein into a living cell and demonstrates that it causes effects characteristic of encephalopathies. Another view of these diseases is that they are caused by virulent strains of extremely stable viruses that resist destruction by common methods and lie hidden within the food being ingested. Thus, these diseases may be caused by a viruslike particle or cofactor that passes on genetic information. This theory would account for the species specificity of these diseases because, as you may remember, many viral diseases have difficulty crossing between species. Thus far, all attempts to find DNA in prions have been unsuccessful. If the prion hypothesis is correct, the fundamental tenet of biology that inheritance passes on from DNA or RNA would have to be reexamined.

THE FAR SIDE   By GARY LARSON

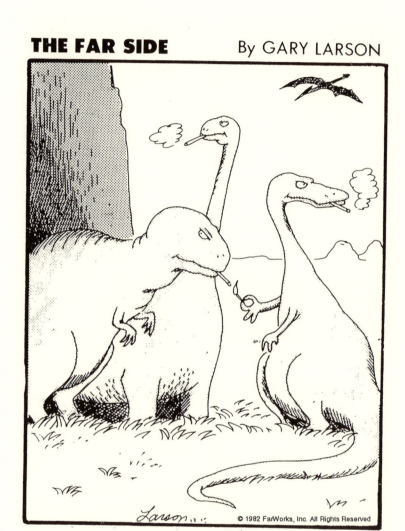

The real reason dinosaurs became extinct.

5

Cancer and the Environment

Cancer and Risk Assessment

Perhaps the most feared of human diseases, cancer is actually a group of diseases caused by the unrestrained growth of cells in one of the body's organs or tissues. Malignant tumors can develop in major organs, such as the lungs, breasts, intestines, skin, stomach, or pancreas, as well as in the blood-forming tissues of the bone marrow (leukemia), and in the lymphatic system. Cancer has affected humans since prehistoric times and is also common in all other animals. Cancer is presently the second most common cause of death in the United States. The public's conception that cancer is unnatural and is principally caused by environmental pollution is the major reason that the public has a fear of chemicals and that many people seek natural cures. Any health measure that increases life expectancy will also drive up the incidence of cancer, as cancer risk increases significantly with age.

Cancer cells have three distinguishing features: (1) they show unregulated growth and proliferation, (2) they have lost the ability to undergo apoptosis, which is programmed cell death, and (3) they are much more susceptible to mutations than normal cells. Mutations appear in cancer cells at a much faster rate than in normal cells. This rapid mutation means that cancer cells are usually heterogeneous— that is, they consist of several kinds of cells—although in a given tumor, all the cancer cells can be traced to a common ancestor cell. The current understanding of all of these problems is still primitive and is under intensive study.

A cancer begins when so-called oncogenes, which are genes that control cell growth and multiplication, are turned on in a cell. Once a cell is transformed into a malignant tumor-forming type, the altered oncogenes are passed on to all offspring cells. This is the way that cells become "immortal." Most cancers are a feature of aging. Both the process of aging and the incidence of cancer can be attributed to accumulated damage to DNA, especially the segments of DNA known as genes, which store information about building enzymes. There are about 30,000 genes in a human; each gene contains the information to synthesize a protein. Many natural agents can damage DNA. Oxygen and oxidants derived from the body's use of oxygen, such as superoxide ion and hydrogen peroxide, are reactive oxidizing agents that attack and alter DNA. It is generally believed that we are protected from DNA damage by antioxidants, such as vitamins C and E and carotene, that we obtain from fruits and vegetables. In 2000, it was surprising to find that these antioxidants may actually nurture the growth of cancer cells, once established. This finding belies Linus Pauling's suggestion that vitamin C should be used to treat cancer patients! Furthermore, beta-carotene supplements have been found not only to be ineffective in protecting against heart disease and cancer, but to actually increase the risk of lung cancer in smokers!

Other cancer-inducing damage to DNA is done by ionizing radiation, such as the ultraviolet component of sunlight or the X-rays that produce the diagnostic images requested by a doctor or dentist. I will discuss such ionizing radiation in more detail later. There are about 60 trillion cells in your body, and about every 10 seconds, every cell, on the average, will take a "hit" from natural or synthetic toxins and from ionizing radiation. As you may already know, cancers are often treated with radiation. It may seem strange that the interaction between radiation and matter that can cause cancer can also be used to kill cancer. This apparent paradox can be understood from the fact that cancer cells divide more rapidly than normal cells, so radiation that damages DNA at the time of cell division is more harmful to the rapidly dividing cancer cells.

Cancers can also be caused by certain viruses that introduce new, harmful sections of their DNA into a cell; the result is a cancer-causing oncogene, which affects growth signals. When a gene that constantly signals growth is encoded into a cell, the cell becomes cancerous and has uncontrolled growth.

Certain classes of chemicals, called carcinogens, also promote cancer. These substances form bonds to the nucleic acid bases in

DNA, leading to mutations. This damage is most dangerous when cells are dividing. The more often cells divide, the shorter the time for the repair machinery to work, and the more likely that a permanent mutation will occur. Thus, processes that stimulate the division of cells are strongly related to human cancers.

Some of the synthetic and naturally occurring chemicals that cause mutations are called alkylating agents. Methyl bromide, a widely used synthetic fungicide, is a good example of such a substance. This simple, volatile chemical is considered essential to the production of strawberries in California, but it may be banned because it helps destroy the ozone layer in the upper atmosphere. Because of its volatility, very little if any methyl bromide ends up in the food chain.

Other carcinogenic compounds are manufactured in our bodies from normally benign chemicals. This sort of transformation is carried out by enzymes in our liver whose job it is to make oily molecules water-soluble by adding oxygen atoms to form alcohol groups. Hydrophobic, polycyclic aromatic hydrocarbons (PAH) in cigarette smoke are transformed into carcinogenic substances in the liver in just this manner; probably some constituents in the smoke of a charcoal barbecue are also turned into carcinogens in our body. Another family of chemical carcinogens, known as heterocyclic amines (HCAs), develop in cooked meats, largely though decomposition of protein. In test-tube experiments, these substances bind to DNA in breast cells, but whether such substances provoke cancer in people is uncertain. Studies of the eating habits of women who did and did not develop breast cancer showed that those who consistently ate meats very well done proved about 4.5 times more likely to have cancer than those who ate rare or medium-cooked meats. Other studies have shown that HCAs develop when meats are cooked at high temperatures for long periods, but not when the meat is seared to a rare state. Curiously, fatty hamburgers developed lower HCA concentrations than lean burgers cooked under the same conditions. These studies are preliminary but counterintuitive; who would have thought rare meat might be safer than well-done meat?

It is interesting that some of the chemicals that are used so successfully to treat cancer, called chemotherapeutic agents, are themselves carcinogens! A more serious problem is that most such drugs are dangerous and lethal at higher-than-recommended doses. Doctors and nurses sometimes make errors, and deaths can result. In one ex-

Cancer and the Environment

ample, patients were given the chemotherapeutic drug Cytoxan (cyclophosphamide) in doses determined according to the patient's body surface area. The correct dosage should have been 1,630 milligrams each day; in one clinic, about four times that amount was given, which proved to be a lethal dose. Overdosing is not an uncommon problem with drugs in general, but it is more serious when it involves the potent chemotherapeutic agents.

Fortunately, we all have hard-working enzymes that repair most of this damage to DNA. Certain classes of enzymes protect us by moving along every strand of DNA, searching for trouble, proofreading our genetic code, and making necessary repairs. These repair enzymes, however, may also be damaged by ionizing radiation or by chemical agents.

You can understand how cancer and aging may be related. Over time, uncorrected damage accumulates; for example, an old rat may have as many as two million DNA lesions. Small animals such as mice and rats have a much higher number of hits to their DNA than humans do. This may explain why rodents live only a few years.

Recent analyses indicate that, despite some press accounts, there is no epidemic of cancer when the current rates are corrected for the effect of smoking and the increased life span of the population. Cancer is a disease of old age, and the population is, on average, getting older. Cancer mortality rates have come down 14% since 1950 (excluding lung cancer, which is largely the result of smoking).

Not all scientists agree. Laurent H. Schwartz, a physician and molecular biologist at the Department of Radiation Therapy at Tenon Hospital in Paris, argues that the incidence of cancer in the United States has increased by 18% since 1981. For example, a European or American woman has a 1 in 11 chance of developing breast cancer during her life. He further argues that surgery is the main key to survival, followed by radiation treatment; anticancer drugs are a distant third. Cancer cells are very "clever" and develop drug resistance that defeats even the most promising chemical and immunotherapeutic treatments. Prevention and early detection are proposed to be the most promising approaches to reducing the effects and mortality of cancer.

Why do some cancers run in families, and why, then, does cancer not develop in every member of such families? Our current understanding of this problem comes from examining the genetic control of cell division. Cancer cells divide without control. The regulation of cell division has been compared to the operation of a car. There are protein growth factors (like a gas pedal) and tumor-suppressing proteins (like a brake). A defective gene may churn out proteins that initiate cell division like a car whose gas pedal is stuck to the floor. Alternatively, the protein that shuts the cell cycle down may not be produced. This is like a failure of the car's brakes. The production of these two types of proteins is controlled by the DNA of the genes. Through mutations, these genes can become defective. Such mutations can be inherited, or they may arise spontaneously when stimulated by environmental factors such as sunlight, naturally occurring chemicals, or just through random mistakes in the normal process of duplicating DNA.

Every gene has two copies of DNA, called alleles; one allele is inherited from each parent for each gene. Each allele carries instructions for producing a particular protein. The two alleles of a gene control the same trait. If, through mutation or inheritance, one allele is defective so that it produces too much of the protein that triggers cell division, like the gas pedal being stuck, the suppressor system may still function (the brakes still work). This type of failure mode is caused by the oncogenes, genes related to cancer. The genes related to your "braking system" have a dual backup, one from each allele. If you inherit one defective gene from your parents, you still have a backup tumor-suppressing protein from the other parent, so you are not doomed to get cancer. If this one good gene becomes damaged by mutation, however, there is no backup. Thus, by inheriting a defective gene, a person has a greater risk of being struck by cancer because they lack a backup gene.

Because of the aging population, within the next two decades cancer is likely to become the leading cause of death in the United States. Cigarette smoking is presently blamed for one-third of all such deaths. Dietary factors have been incriminated in another third, but the details are uncertain. Viruses and bacteria are thought to account for more than 15% of cancers in developing countries but perhaps less in the United States. Examples are hepatitis virus (liver cancer), herpes virus (Kaposi's sarcoma), papilloma viruses (cervical cancer), and the helical bacterium that causes stomach cancer. On the other hand, environmental pollution from occupational exposure is thought to cause perhaps 5% of cancers, and only 2% is considered to be caused by environmental pollutants. Some people argue, however, that these latter two numbers should be much higher.

The Delaney clause

In 1958, a very stringent regulation was introduced that ruled illegal in foods *any* synthetic substance that is *claimed* to cause cancer in *any test animal* at *any level* of application. At the time, cancer was considered the most important disease threat, few carcinogens were recognized, and routine analytical methods were crude. Ruling out any detectable pesticide residue seemed reasonable at that time. As analytical methods have become ever more powerful, the Delaney law seems to be ever more foolish. Modern instruments can detect residues at a femtogram level (10^{-15} of 1 gram). The biological meaning of such a tiny quantity is not clear; what can a femtogram of a carcinogen do? In 1996, the Delaney clause was modified, and a new standard for evaluating the health and safety of pesticides was established in its place. This standard uses a "reasonable certainty of no harm." The evaluation of these substances is still controversial, however.

What is wrong with these precautions? Bruce Ames (of the University of California, Berkeley) and many other scientists now believe that megadoses of anything that can accelerate cell division can lead to cancer. Furthermore, using the test he invented, Ames has found huge numbers of naturally occurring pesticides in food. As he states, "Almost every plant product in the supermarket is likely to contain natural carcinogens." Half of all chemicals tested in high doses on animals, whether natural or synthetic, are carcinogens. One problem with the Delaney clause is that the high-test-dose effect may not be relevant at low doses. Plants make their own insecticides. Of 64 natural plant pesticides that have been tested, 35 are carcinogens! For example, more than 1,000 chemicals have been reported in roasted coffee; 26 have been tested, and 19 have been found to be carcinogens. Each day, on average, every American eats a gram and a half of such natural pesticides; this is more than 10,000 times higher than the residues ingested from man-made agricultural pesticides. Forty-three foods were determined to contain at least 10 parts per million of chemicals that were determined to be carcinogenic in high-dose rodent tests. These foods include many familiar items: parsley, oregano, sage, rosemary, and thyme.

Recall that all animals (like us) have natural defense mechanisms to fight damage to our DNA. You might ask whether we are wasting much of the estimated $150 billion spent each year trying to control pollution. Although some of this activity is clearly desirable, this exceptional expenditure may have little influence on cancer rates. We spend 100 times more trying to save a life by attempting to intercept a suspected toxin than we do trying to improve a medical intervention. Also, the money spent on biomedical research is minimal compared with the costs of implementing and complying with Environmental Protection Agency regulations. In my opinion more attention should be paid to well-known, real dangers such as smoking and lack of proper diet. Remember that the major causes of cancer are thought to be smoking (about one-third), lack of dietary fruits and vegetables, and chronic infections (mostly in developing nations). Epidemiologic studies show that the most effective ways to reduce cancer risk are by not smoking, avoiding direct sunlight, and eating fresh fruits and vegetables.

Next, you may wonder if the body has any other mechanisms to protect itself against cancer. It does: the immune system.

The Immune System: Jekyll And Hyde

Your immune system is your natural defense against bacterial and viral infections and against cancer. This system can be prepared to attack a particular invader by vaccination. It is the principal defense you have against viruses, and it can also ward off some bacteria. Our immune defense can become our enemy, however, and it can cause many ailments broadly referred to as autoimmune diseases. Various forms of arthritis are caused by the immune system's mistaking one's own cells as enemies and destroying tissues in the body. You may be interested in some of the science behind the immune system.

Mammals are able to recognize individual cells in their bodies as being either "foreign" or "self." The cells associated with this defense network are largely found in the blood and may be familiar to you. The most important immune system cells are called B and T cells (the letters stand for bone marrow and thymus, respectively). The B cells produce antibodies, which are protein molecules that bind to foreign cells and mark them for destruction by other components of the immune system. There are different types of T cells that have many roles; an important type is the killer T cells that destroy foreign cells. T-cell-mediated immunity requires at least two cells to recognize a foreign cell. This type of defense serves as a safety device to prevent the immune system from attacking the body's normal cells.

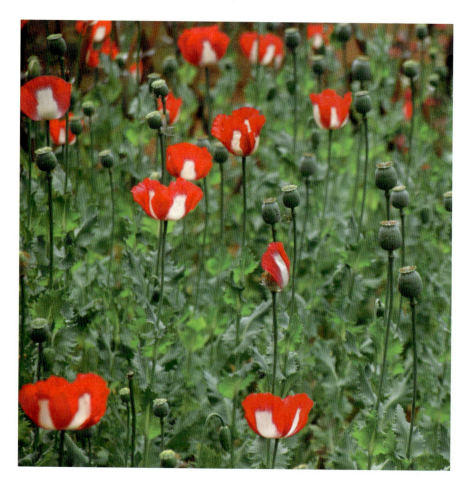

Figure 5. The opium poppy from which opium is obtained.

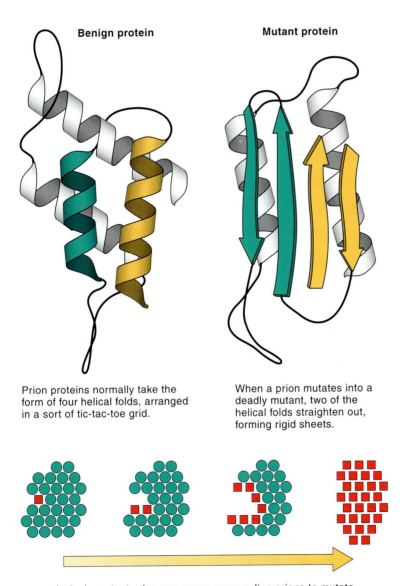

Benign protein

Mutant protein

Prion proteins normally take the form of four helical folds, arranged in a sort of tic-tac-toe grid.

When a prion mutates into a deadly mutant, two of the helical folds straighten out, forming rigid sheets.

A single mutant prion can cause surrounding prions to mutate. These, in turn, infect adjacent prions in a snowball effect.

Figure 7. A proposed transformation of a benign prion protein into a mutant form.

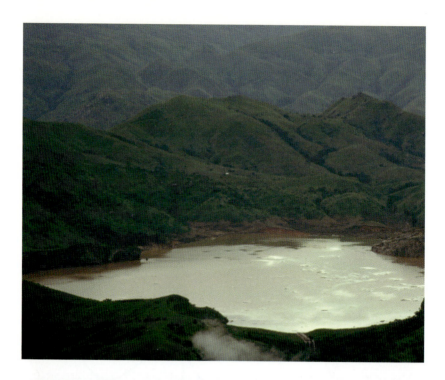

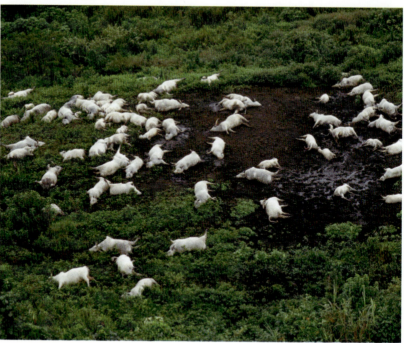

Figure 10. In 1986 Lake Nyos in Cameroon (top) released a huge bubble of CO_2, suffocating people and animals living nearby (bottom).

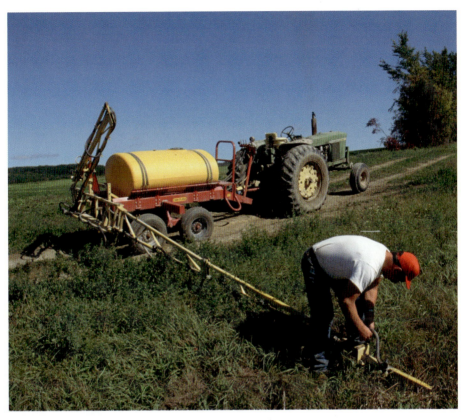

Figure 11. A farmer is preparing to inject liquefied ammonia (NH_3) directly into the soil as a fertilizer.

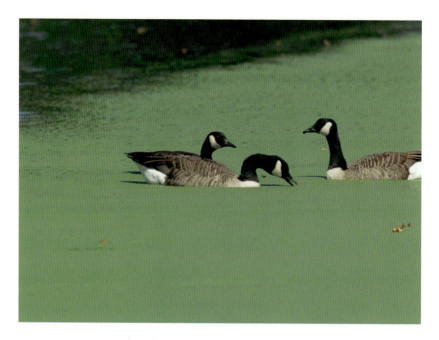

Figure 12. Algae blooms caused by phosphate pollution.

Figure 16. Trees damaged by acid rain.

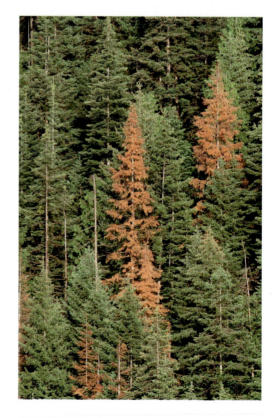

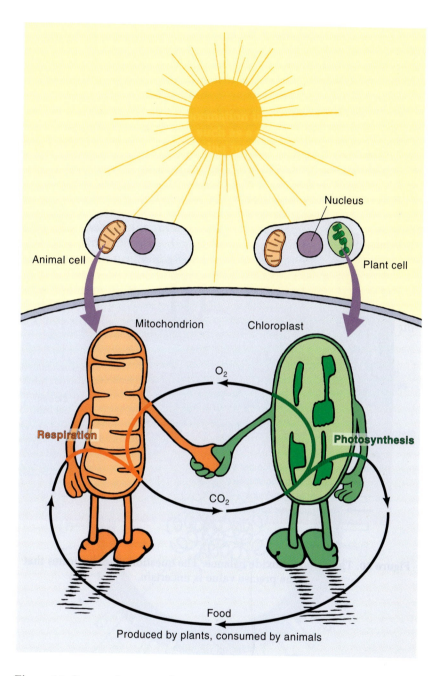

Figure 19. Synergy between photosynthesis (in chloroplasts) and respiration (in mitochondria) is responsible for the balance of carbon dioxide (CO_2) and oxygen (O_2) on Earth. Plants and algae use energy from sunlight to convert CO_2 into energy-rich substances (food) with concomitant release of a by-product (O_2). The latter is used by most organisms, including mammals, to oxidize foods, producing energy that sustains life, and to regenerate CO_2.

portant to understand that immunological encounters do not become genetically inscribed and passed on to future generations. Some immunity may be passed from a mother to her child through nursing and by contact with others in a community, but it is not an inherited trait.

Although the immune system may have memory cells to fight reinfection by a particular virus, recall that the virus can undergo mutation; thus, the immune system may not recognize a modified virus. This is one reason you have to be inoculated against new forms of influenza virus every year. Immunization is the main line of defense against viral infections, but, as mentioned earlier, it is not very effective against the rapidly mutating retroviruses such as the human immunodeficiency virus (HIV), the virus that causes AIDS. Because of the rapid mutation of retroviruses, it is very difficult to develop effective vaccines against them.

This technique of vaccination has been practiced since 1796, when Edward Jenner reported that inoculating people with material from a cowpox sore would protect them from the more dangerous smallpox. The explorers Lewis and Clark took a crude smallpox vaccine on their epic expedition, with instructions to inoculate Indians along the way. At various times in history, vaccination was considered a miracle preventative technique that protected the general public against terrible, often deadly diseases, but at present, the general public is forgetting and foregoing this important public health defense. Older people may vividly recall the terror of polio, but young parents have no personal memory of this. Many people do not know the terrors of whooping cough, of potentially fatal throat infections from diphtheria, and of measles that can result in mental retardation. This lack of personal experience and ignorance of the dangers has led to a disturbing complacency among some parents about protecting infants against dangerous, infectious diseases through vaccination. All 50 states require vaccinations before a child may enter school, but many preschoolers are left unprotected, especially in poor, minority communities.

By this point, you have learned that nothing is completely safe, and that is also true of vaccination. A vaccine called DPT, for diphtheria, pertussis, and tetanus, has, in rare instances, caused seizures and brain damage in small children. The vaccine has since been improved, but there is still a small risk, so some parents resist having their children vaccinated. They believe there is no danger because these diseases are rare and the presence of the other, vaccinated children will protect their own, unvaccinated youngsters. This concept is called *herd immunity,* but it is a dangerous one. A few years ago, when 75% of children were vaccinated against measles, some other, unvaccinated children got the disease, and some died. A few people who believe in "natural medicines" and avoid antibiotics and other modern medicines are also opposed to vaccination. They should read the following historical account of diseases, from before and after the time when people could get vaccinated and thereby protected from viral diseases such as smallpox. In the late 1970s, this once-dreaded scourge became the first disease to be eradicated from the human experience.

Examples of the Role of Microorganisms and the Immune System in History

Before vaccination was developed, another method called variolation was used to immunize people by inoculating them with live infectious material taken from a living patient who had smallpox. Variolation is a more hazardous preventive measure than vaccination, but it is better than receiving no treatment. This technique had an important and controversial role in the American Revolutionary War. In 1771, a smallpox epidemic occurred in Boston, and inoculation there was promoted by a clergyman named Mather and a surgeon named Boylston; it was opposed, however, by a Scottish doctor named Douglass. The selectmen in Boston rejected the public-health use of inoculation. Some Boston citizens opposed to inoculation threw a lighted hand grenade into Mather's room as a part of their protest. In 1775, George Washington, the new commander of the Colonial Army, ordered the inoculation of his army and all recruits to control the smallpox epidemic among his troops. The British commander, Howe, did not address the issue of smallpox. Howe's withdrawal from Boston may have been caused by a smallpox epidemic that broke out among his troops. Washington's controversial variolation program is believed to have contributed significantly to the winning of independence by the colonies. Today, the dangerous variolation method is permitted only on nonhumans.

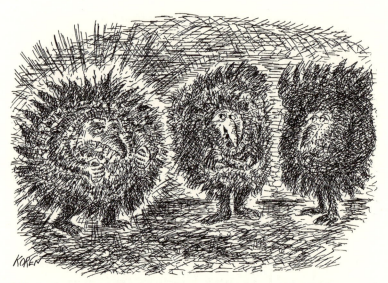

"She's the most effective of our emerging new pathogens."

The role of lethal microbes in human history is best illustrated by Europeans' conquest and depopulation of the New World. Many more Native Americans died of European-borne infections than of attack by European guns and swords. Deadly plagues occur when microorganisms are introduced into a population that has no immunity. In the history of humankind, the vulnerability of isolated populations against a new infectious agent has resulted in many important historical changes. You may wonder why isolated populations are so sensitive to new microorganisms.

Long association with a particular virus or bacterium leads to the evolution of some degree of immunity in a population, but a group that has never encountered these infectious agents has no defense. In the years following the Spanish conquest and in the invasion of the American West by trappers and explorers, common European diseases such as measles, influenza, and smallpox killed large numbers of native peoples in the Americas. For example, in 1518, Cortez invaded what is now Mexico. From then through 1595, a series of diseases—smallpox, mumps, and measles, which were previously un-

Table 7   Deadly "Gifts" from Our Domesticated Animal Friends[a]

Human disease	Animal with most closely related pathogen
Measles	Cattle (rinderpest)
Tuberculosis	Cattle
Smallpox	Cattle (cowpox) or other livestock with related pox viruses
Influenza	Pigs, ducks
Pertussis	Pigs, dogs
Falciparum malaria	Birds (chicken and ducks?)

[a]Adapted from Diamond, F. 1999. *Guns, germs, and steel: The fates of human societies.* New York: W. W. Norton.

known in the Americas—resulted in the death of 18.5 million of the total population of 25 million people.

Where did these human infectious agents originate? It is believed that agricultural populations were first exposed to viruses from their domesticated animals and thus developed some immunity to these pathogens. In contrast, hunters and gatherers possessed few domestic animals and were more susceptible to these microorganisms when they came in contact with more civilized peoples. This theory would account for the extreme sensitivity that isolated peoples such as Native Americans, Hawaiians, and Australian Aborigines showed toward invaders. Table 7 lists some common diseases that are thought to have originated in domesticated animals. One can speculate that this problem could account for the demise of the ancient hominids, the Neanderthals, a hunter–gatherer group, when they encountered early modern humans, who had domesticated animals.

This same phenomenon can occur whenever domestic animals come into contact with populations of wild animals. In 1994, domestic canine distemper, a virus related to measles, killed 1,000 lions—one-third of the population in the Serengeti National Park in Tanzania. This situation, which has been repeated in many parts of the world, is a threat to some of the rarest wild animals.

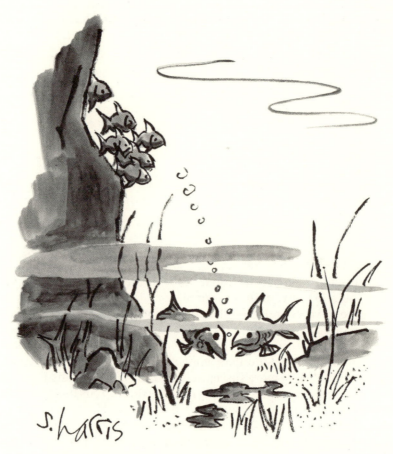

"THE DEVIL WITH THE FOOD CHAIN.
I LIKE MERCURY."

6

Nature Is Elemental

MANY PEOPLE ARE FRIGHTENED of chemicals, but what *are* chemicals? Simply defined, chemicals are materials made from the elements found in the periodic table, which is essentially a map of the elements. You will discover that some elements or simple compounds derived from these elements are required for life but may be dangerous in certain circumstances. Other elements are toxic. I begin with examples from the first column of elements on the left side of the periodic table (Figure 9). In their elemental (metallic) form, these elements react violently with water or air. In nature, these elements are never found in the metallic state but rather as positively charged atoms called cations in salts.

Metals

Lithium

The lithium cation is not required for life, but it was discovered (by chance) to be efficacious in the treatment of bipolar (manic-depressive) mental illness. Lithium is administered prophylactically as lithium carbonate. Although this medicine is very effective, there is a problem: slightly higher concentrations of lithium cations are *toxic*! This is another encounter with a common theme: a little of something is good or necessary, but more may be dangerous. Patients receiving lithium carbonate therapy must have their blood levels monitored for the concentration of lithium cations; this analysis is difficult and complicates the use of this therapy.

121

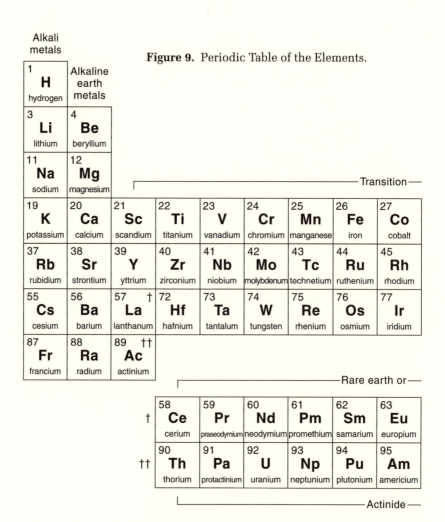

Figure 9. Periodic Table of the Elements.

Sodium and potassium

The sodium cation is required for life, and it is usually ingested as table salt, sodium chloride. The human body needs about 200 mg of sodium chloride per day (roughly the amount in one-tenth of a teaspoon of salt). Sodium regulates vital functions such as muscle movement, blood pressure, and nerve impulses. Most people consume far more salt than they require (15 to 20 times more); most

Nature is Elemental

Noble
gases

Halogens

									Noble gases

Boundary line between metals and nonmetals

metals

			5 **B** boron	6 **C** carbon	7 **N** nitrogen	8 **O** oxygen	9 **F** fluorine	10 **Ne** neon
			13 **Al** aluminum	14 **Si** silicon	15 **P** phosphorus	16 **S** sulfur	17 **Cl** chlorine	18 **Ar** argon
28 **Ni** nickel	29 **Cu** copper	30 **Zn** zinc	31 **Ga** gallium	32 **Ge** germanium	33 **As** arsenic	34 **Se** selenium	35 **Br** bromine	36 **Kr** krypton
46 **Pd** palladium	47 **Ag** silver	48 **Cd** cadmium	49 **In** indium	50 **Sn** tin	51 **Sb** antimony	52 **Te** tellurium	53 **I** iodine	54 **Xe** xenon
78 **Pt** platinum	79 **Au** gold	80 **Hg** mercury	81 **Tl** thallium	82 **Pb** lead	83 **Bi** bismuth	84 **Po** polonium	85 **At** astatine	86 **Rn** radon

lanthanide metals

64 **Gd** gadolinium	65 **Tb** terbium	66 **Dy** dysprosium	67 **Ho** holmium	68 **Er** erbium	69 **Tm** thulium	70 **Yb** ytterbium	71 **Lu** lutetium
96 **Cm** curium	97 **Bk** berkelium	98 **Cf** californium	99 **Es** einsteinium	100 **Fm** fermium	101 **Md** mendelevium	102 **No** nobelium	103 **Lr** lawrencium

metals

eliminate this excess in their urine. However, 30% to 50% of hypertensive patients (those with high blood pressure) cannot efficiently eliminate this excess salt. These individuals are subject to serious medical problems caused by excess sodium ions; these problems include stroke, congestive heart failure, pulmonary edema (buildup of excess fluid in the lungs), osteoporosis in postmenopausal women, a higher incidence of stomach cancer, and kidney disease. Too much salt also seems to deplete calcium levels in the bone. The potential dangers of excess salt consumption by the general public are somewhat controversial, however.

High concentrations of the sodium cation are found in many processed foods as sodium chloride. These include sausages, corned beef, hot dogs, smoked fish, most dry cereals, soups, salad dressing, mustard, most cheeses, chips, and pretzels! Many of these are foods we all like and consume. The health threat of excess salt consumption is a classic toxic problem—a little is vital to life, but more may be quite hazardous, depending on the individual.

Potassium is also essential for life. Because it is similar to sodium, potassium chloride is sometimes used as a salt substitute. When potassium is used in excess, this essential element can be harmful to people with kidney problems and to those taking certain heart-failure medications and diuretics. Besides, potassium chloride does not taste very good! Potassium is also interesting because it is a source of little-recognized radioactivity in our bodies! A rare radioactive isotope, ^{40}K, is present in all potassium (0.00118%). On average, adults have about 150 grams of potassium dissolved in their body fluids. All of our food contains some potassium. Therefore, you are radioactive and consume radioactive food whether you like it or not. Not to worry, there is not much radioactive potassium around; a small enough amount of anything is probably not dangerous. We will return to this point.

Beryllium, magnesium, and calcium

Adjacent to sodium and potassium in the periodic table are elements normally existing as doubly charged cations. The lightest of these elements, beryllium, is *highly toxic.* You never encounter beryllium in foods, but it is sometimes present in electrical equipment and as an alloy in bearings. Care must be taken in disposing of these products.

The next two very similar elements, magnesium and calcium, are required for life in their 2^+ cation (dication) forms. Much of your skeleton and teeth are composed of calcium phosphate. These dications are essential for cell function; a deficiency of calcium is involved in osteoporosis. Calcium ions have many biological roles in sugar metabolism, muscle contraction, and vision. Calcium deficiency can be avoided by consuming food products such as milk, yogurt, cheese, sardines, and soy products, all of which are rich in calcium.

Calcium phosphate is quite insoluble; a common form of kidney stones contains calcium phosphate crystals. Excess dietary calcium intake is not considered to be the source of kidney-stone formation, but dehydration is. Deposits of another insoluble salt, calcium oxalate, are found in kidney stones and in certain forms of gout. Magnesium and calcium ions themselves are not considered toxic, but one could probably take a toxic overdose of their salts. In 1995, it was reported that excessive consumption of antacid medication can raise a person's magnesium levels, causing stomach aches and kidney problems.

Chromium

Chromium is a so-called transition metal; it may be found in the chrome-plated bumper of your car. A derivative of chromium, the chromate anion, is a carcinogen. A commonly encountered 3^+ chromium ion has been used for many years in leather tanning, and toxic chromium wastes from the leather industries contaminate several streams in Europe. Chromium salts can be purchased in health food stores as a mineral supplement; many people take chromium supplements. Why? Chromium is claimed to be an essential element, required in trace amounts for carbohydrate metabolism. Plants such as shepherd's purse that accumulate chromium have been used as a folk medicine to treat diabetes, but no careful study of this herbal remedy appears to exist.

Small quantities of chromium are found in several foods, including liver, cheese, whole-grain breads and cereals, beans, yeast, and vegetables such as broccoli. Animals who are fed a completely chromium-free diet become very ill. However, a diet containing anything more than trace amounts of chromium salts may be dangerous! Chromium is an example of an element that is claimed to be required for life in tiny amounts but is toxic in larger amounts, especially in particular forms.

Chromium picolinate is a widely sold dietary supplement used by fitness buffs, people trying to lose weight, and others who frequent health food stores. The recommended daily intake for adults is only 50 to 200 micrograms (less than a small grain of salt). This chromium derivative is able to penetrate the cell's genetic machinery and may damage chromosomes. Such damage is an indicator of cancer-causing potential. More research needs to be done before this supplement can be considered safe. Preliminary studies at the University of Dayton in

Ohio found that a chromium-fortified drink boosted by 7% the sprint performance of cyclists over that of a placebo. The risk–benefit analysis of chromium supplements will require extensive studies.

Iron

Iron is an excellent example of an element necessary for life at one concentration and life threatening at another. The situation depends on the individual and his or her sex! Iron deficiency is uncommon. Only about 5% of premenopausal women, 2% of postmenopausal women, and 1% of men actually have iron deficiency, or anemia. These individuals can increase their iron levels by taking iron supplements and eating red meat. Vegetarians can usually get enough iron by eating iron-rich plant foods such as legumes, dark-green leafy vegetables, and fortified breads.

Too much iron in the body can create excess free radicals, the potentially destructive molecules that are implicated in a wide range of diseases. Iron is also involved in the formation of plaque deposits, which can clog arteries. About 1 person in 250 has a genetic disorder called hemochromatosis that results in extremely high iron levels. These individuals have an increased risk of developing liver cancer, heart disease, diabetes, impotence, and arthritis! Even people who don't have hemochromatosis may show moderately high iron levels and have some increased risk of heart disease and cancer. People with high iron levels are advised to avoid taking iron supplements, limit their consumption of red meat (which is rich in iron), and exercise regularly, because that helps lower iron stores. Donating blood also helps decrease amount of iron in the body. A British study published in 1997 reported that men who had given at least a pint of blood every 3 years were 30% less likely to suffer a heart attack or stroke, undergo heart surgery, or require heart medications than men who had not given blood. Women lose blood through menstruation and have about half the risk of cardiovascular disease as men. This association between the iron levels and cardiovascular diseases may be incidental. More research is needed on this question.

Cobalt

Cobalt is the transition element that gives the blue color to "cobalt glass"; it is also essential for life. To be effective, cobalt must be ingested as a macrocyclic complex (similar to, but not quite the same as, the iron complex in hemoglobin or the magnesium-containing green photosynthetic pigment, chlorophyll). This cobalt complex is vitamin B_{12}. This vitamin must be ingested intact because it cannot be synthesized by animals or plants—vitamin B_{12} is produced only by certain microorganisms! Without ingesting any vitamin B_{12}, you would get pernicious anemia (low red blood cell count). A healthy person requires very little of this vitamin per day (less than a tiny grain of salt, about 10^{-5} g). Meats—especially liver—provide ample vitamin B_{12}, but plants do not. Rarely do people suffer from a dietary shortage of B_{12}—only very strict vegetarians, who are advised to take vitamin B_{12} supplements. Ingestion of megadoses of vitamin B_{12} is dangerous, however.

Simple cobalt salts are toxic! Several years ago, a Canadian beer poisoned some individuals because of inadvertent contamination with cobalt salts. With cobalt, we again find that a little is essential (in this case in a specific form), and a lot can be deadly.

Copper

Although large quantities of copper are toxic, copper is essential to biological function. Many copper-bearing enzymes are involved in reactions involving oxygen, such as respiration. Copper is essential in an important enzyme, cytochrome c oxidase, which is required to generate energy in the body.

The recommended daily intake of dietary copper is 2 to 3 mg (equivalent to about two small grains of salt). The typical US diet may be deficient in copper. Foods rich in copper are calf liver, crabs, certain cereals, nuts, and cocoa. Too much copper in the body is toxic. The body's ability to utilize copper varies with age and amount of exercise. The elderly sometimes absorb less copper and its companion metal, zinc. Aerobic exercise elevates copper and zinc levels in the blood serum of 60- to 80-year-old patients. Studies of rats fed copper-deficient diets showed elevated levels of copper after they drank beer, which contains only trace amounts of copper. Beer may enhance the utilization of copper—at least in rats! On the other hand, the types of dietary fiber that bring about certain positive effects, such as lowering cholesterol, act to *decrease* the utilization of minerals, including copper. The best nutritional advice is to eat a balanced diet of conventional food.

Zinc

Near copper in the periodic table is zinc, another essential element that is found at the active site in several enzymes. Zinc has many biochemical roles, some of which are not well understood. Zinc supplements of about 25 mg (approximately one-quarter of a small aspirin tablet) are recommended for thin, pregnant women, who are typically zinc deficient. Zinc deficiencies can result in undersized fetuses. Male fertility and potency are enhanced by zinc. (Perhaps this is why Casanova ate so many oysters, which are rich in zinc.) Zinc also enhances the sensation of taste. Zinc deficiency can result in a serious, congenital eye disease, macular degeneration, which results in loss of sight at the center of the eye.

Too much zinc can be deleterious, however. Zinc supplements raise levels of LDL (the "bad" cholesterol), lower those of HDL (the "good" cholesterol), and remove the beneficial effects of exercise on HDL levels. A preliminary report from Australia suggests that zinc supplements initiate an Alzheimerlike condition in elderly patients. Zinc is not highly toxic and is required, but it should be consumed in moderate quantities. Perhaps it is better to avoid zinc supplements, even though these are popular with certain health faddists.

Aluminum

The toxicity of aluminum is controversial. Some scientists claim that the brains of diseased Alzheimer's patients contain significantly more aluminum than those from other patients. Others dispute this claim and argue that the presence of this metal in senile plaques is incidental or occurred after death. Aluminum in the brain would interfere with DNA in nerve cells, acting as Crazy Glue would to the pages of a book. A protein, transferrin, binds aluminum in the blood and may keep it out of the brain. Early dialysis machines introduced toxic levels of aluminum into patients, but that is no longer a problem. In the past, some people avoided cooking with aluminum pots. I find the little-known presence of aluminum salts in some baking powders to be unnecessary. Probably you have ingested aluminum derived from this source.

Lead

In contrast to sodium, potassium, magnesium, calcium, cobalt, copper, and zinc, which are essential to life at some level, lead is a bad metal to introduce into your body. Although toxic, lead has many useful, nonbiological properties. Lead has been used in plumbing from ancient times to the present. Some lead pipes installed by the Romans are still in use today. The peak Roman use, 2,000 years ago, is estimated to have been 80,000 tons per year.

Lead is also used in glass (in wine decanters and goblets), in pottery, in automobile batteries, and as a gasoline "antiknock" agent (tetraethyllead). An advertisement from a national retail store suggested people might have been poisoned by chewing on pencils. This misinformation amused my students, who know that the "lead" in pencils is actually graphite (a form of carbon).

People vary greatly in their susceptibility to lead poisoning; children and fetuses are much more sensitive, and the metal can lead to learning disorders. The body excretes lead at a moderate rate (it has a half-life of about three weeks), but lead accumulates in bone (and in baby teeth). Except for damage to children, there is no general agreement about this metal's health effects at low levels. Lead poisoning is thought by some to have contributed to the fall of Rome. One of the ancient Romans' more insidious exposures to lead came from their use of a red paste ("sapa") made from boiling down spoiled wine in lead pots. We now know that sapa is lead acetate. The Romans used sapa because it is sweet. Their supply of honey was insufficient (sugar was not yet known), and Roman cooks used sapa as an artificial sweetener in as many as 85 recipes. It is now thought that sapa may have contributed to the reputed infertility of the Roman upper class. Roman prostitutes were especially fond of sapa; it served as a method of birth control and lightened their skin tone (as it probably also shortened their lives). Lead acetate, called sugar of lead, was still used as a sweetener through the 1800s. In those times, vintners added lead shot to port wine to increase its sweetness.

Recently, the allowable concentrations of lead have been limited by the US Occupational Safety and Health Administration (OSHA). In drinking water, a limit of 50 parts per billion (ppb) allowed in 1977 was reduced to 15 ppb in 1991. In 1995, the workplace threshold limit value for airborne lead was reduced to 0.05 mg per cubic meter (5 ppb). The use of lead in paint was banned by federal law in 1978, after a slow phase-out. Lead is being phased out of gasoline for a reason other than its human toxicity. Lead poisons the automobile exhaust catalysts that reduce air pollution. As the result of these controls, the average blood-lead levels in the United States have fallen 78% to 2.8 mg/dl—a very low level.

There are other avenues by which people can be exposed to lead. For example, individuals can be exposed from using leaded glass, such as crystal decanters. A sample of brandy stored in a lead-glass crystal decanter was found to have a lead concentration more than 400 times the threshold for lead poisoning in a person's blood. Another source is lead foil, which has been used to seal wine bottles. To avoid contamination, it is recommended that after removing the cork, the spout of the wine bottle should be wiped off before pouring the wine. A British study found the first glass of wine poured from an unwiped bottle had 320 parts per billion (ppb) of lead; even after wiping off the bottle before pouring, the lead reading was 250 ppb. Red wine stored in such a bottle was found to have an "acceptable" level of lead (57 ppb). The traditional lead foil over the cork on wine bottles is being phased out in the United States because of concerns over lead toxicity. Some modern wines, such as those from the Robert Mondavi Winery in California, are now covered with a new beeswax seal in place of the lead foil.

Mercury

Mercury is widespread; it is not essential to life, but we are all exposed to this toxic element. Even in ancient times, mercury was known to be toxic. The Roman naturalist and writer Pliny the Elder described the high mortality rate of workers in mercury mines. The expression "mad as a hatter" derived from the psychological disturbances as well as swollen gums and tremors in the hands of workers in the felt-hat industry. Felt was made by treating fur with acidic solutions of mercury nitrate. Dicationic mercury is known to be toxic; the tiny felt particles carried these mercury salts into the hatter's body. The toxicity of mercury depends on its chemical state and the nature of the exposure. For example, metallic mercury was drunk as a laxative in the Middle Ages; mercury dental amalgam is widely used today. There is no evidence that either practice is dangerous, even though drinking metallic mercury seems ridiculous today.

Mercury metal is a volatile liquid; it has a measurable vapor pressure at room temperature. This means that in a room where mercury metal drops are exposed to the air, mercury atoms are present in that air. Inhalation of the mercury vapor is considered toxic to the lungs. About 3,500 tons of mercury is spewed out in the world each year, largely from burning coal, oil, and wood (60%), and from waste incineration (36%). Mercury enters our waterways from many sources.

One important source of mercury pollution is being phased out—the electrochemical production of chlorine (Cl_2) once used mercury electrode cells. In the 1980s, about 1 million pounds of mercury was released into US waters as a result of chlorine production.

Bacteria present in sludge, river sediment, and the ocean convert mercury metal and mercuric ions into monomethylmercury derivatives and into dimethylmercury; the latter two substances are very dangerous. These nonpolar compounds have carbon–mercury bonds and are soluble in fat. As hydrophobic compounds, they become concentrated in the fatty tissue of fish, especially in the liver. Fish living in a mercury-polluted lake may have a mercury concentration thousands of times that of the water they live in. Health authorities must test the fish, not the water, to determine safety. In humans, these fat-soluble compounds find their way to the brain, where they can cause neurologic damage.

An example of this phenomenon of mercury poisoning through fish consumption is the Minamata Bay disaster in Japan, which resulted in many deaths and numerous cases of brain damage between 1948 and 1960 from the consumption of mercury-laden fish. In fact, millions of fish lovers today do have low levels of mercury in their bodies. People who eat whale meat have somewhat higher levels than eaters of fish because the whales, being higher in the ocean food chain, concentrate mercury from the smaller creatures they eat. The World Health Organization suggests a maximum mercury concentration of 10 parts per million in the hair, which is a measure of mercury in the human body. A study of children in the Faroe Islands, where pilot whales are widely consumed, showed a correlation of mercury levels in children with lower mental performance, including problems with learning, attention, memory, and other mental skills. According to the study, the more mercury the children had, the more poorly they performed. This result has led some to call for lowering allowable exposure to mercury by perhaps tenfold. An analysis balancing the benefits of fish consumption against the danger of mercury exposure within the United States concludes that reduction of coronary heart disease outweighs the lower risks from mercury exposure, with the possible exception of young children and pregnant women. Fish are useful as direct dietary sources of beneficial omega-3 polyunsaturated fatty acids, which are important for brain and retinal development, motor development, and the duration of sleep in human infants.

Mercury concentration in the hair of Seychelle Islands population is, on average, 10 to 20 times the average in the United States because the Seychellois consume about 12 fish meals per week. Any potential adverse effects of mercury consumption should be detected in the Seychelles population long before such effects would be seen in the United States. The eating of fish and possible exposure to mercury is a classic case of risk versus benefit.

The highly toxic, fat-soluble compound dimethylmercury is especially dangerous because it is quite volatile and can penetrate latex rubber gloves and a person's skin. In 1997, a Dartmouth University chemistry professor, Karen Wetterman, died after she worked with this substance in a fume hood while wearing rubber gloves. She suffered severe neurologic damage. Until recently, this dangerous mercury compound could be sent through the mail! A related, less dangerous, but still toxic mercury compound, phenylmercury acetate, was once used as a fungicide in seed corn, which was not intended to be eaten. Some poor children in New Mexico did eat such seed corn and died as a result. This same substance was once sold as a fungicide in swimming pool stores. How many readers have been exposed to tiny amounts of this agent in swimming pools? Both uses have since ceased because of concerns over toxicity.

Around 1990, there was widespread public alarm about the use of mercury in dental fillings. The typical composition of traditional dental amalgams is: mercury, 50%; silver, 35%; tin, 13%; copper, 1.55%; zinc, 0.5%. Even though no epidemiologic evidence showed impaired health from these amalgams, many people became so alarmed that they had all of their fillings drilled out (ugh!) and replaced with gold or plastic! In 1991, a scientific panel convened by the National Institutes of Health to study this question concluded that "there is no scientific evidence that dental fillings containing mercury cause significant adverse side effects." The hysteria over this issue has largely died out in the United States, but in 1998, it resurfaced in New Zealand.

There are some medicinal uses of mercury compounds; perhaps you remember mercurochrome, a not very effective antibacterial agent used for minor abrasions. Thimerosal is used as a topical antiseptic and preservative in eye drops; it is an ethylmercury derivative bound to a sulfur group (mercury has a very high affinity for sulfur). These agents should not be imbibed or introduced into a deep cut. Calomel is a derivative of mercury in the 1^+ state that was once used as a laxative. This application is still permitted, but such use is rare. One danger is that decomposition of calomel can result in toxic 2^+

mercuric ions. In summary, mercury is a widespread metal that is very toxic in some forms, especially within the body, but in other forms and in other applications mercury is not especially dangerous.

Thallium

Thallium is toxic in all forms—the metal, the 1^+ cation, and the 3^+ cation. For this reason, every effort should be made to keep thallium out of the biosphere. It has been used as rat poison.

Nonmetallic Elements

Nonmetallic elements are found on the right side of the periodic table. They tend to take up (attract and keep) electrons, thereby forming negatively charged atoms called anions; alternatively, they form strong bonds with other elements. Both the toxic and benign properties of some nonmetallic elements and their compounds illustrate the same principles you have seen for metallic elements: the form and the amount of an element are what determines whether that element is toxic.

Boron

Compounds of boron such as borax are used as cleansers; in large quantities, however, borax is toxic and has been forbidden in foods for about 50 years by the US Food and Drug Administration. In some other parts of the world, borax is sometimes added to caviar because it makes the caviar sweeter and gives it a better texture. Most of us need not worry about poisoning ourselves by overeating caviar; the best stuff, Beluga caviar, ranges from $300 to $800 for 14 ounces! You will not find a borax additive listed on the label.

Carbon

The branches of chemistry known as organic and biological chemistry concern compounds of carbon. Here, I will consider only two molecules that contain carbon. The first is a toxic chemical that you may recognize because it is often in the news—carbon monoxide (CO). It is important to distinguish carbon monoxide from the second molecule, the nontoxic gas carbon dioxide (CO_2), which occurs naturally in the atmosphere and is an exhaust product from combustion and respiration.

Carbon monoxide is a colorless, odorless gas that binds to iron in the hemoglobin of your blood, thereby preventing the iron atom from carrying oxygen. All air-breathing (aerobic) creatures are subject to carbon monoxide poisoning. Carbon monoxide results from incomplete combustion; your automobile exhaust contains some carbon monoxide (less if fitted with a catalytic converter); charcoal grills give off large quantities of carbon monoxide. That is why either source can kill you in a confined, unventilated space. A running car in a closed garage is a familiar method of suicide—in fiction and in real life. Occasionally, someone is sufficiently ignorant or careless to operate a charcoal grill indoors. Carbon monoxide detectors are widely marketed; some government agencies require installation of such detectors in apartments and office buildings. Did you know that you could set off a very sensitive carbon monoxide detector by just breathing on it?! How can this be so? The reason is that your body constantly gives off carbon monoxide as it degrades compounds called porphyrins from your hemoglobin. As a result, you exhale small amounts of carbon monoxide; its concentration in your blood is about three parts per million. Oxygen in higher concentrations can compete with carbon monoxide. The oxygen and carbon monoxide molecules line up to bind to the hemoglobin in your blood. If there are many more oxygen than carbon monoxide molecules, they win, even though carbon monoxide molecules bind more tenaciously. That is why smokers are not killed outright by the carbon monoxide formed by their burning cigarettes, although carbon monoxide and other combustion products have other long-term, toxic effects.

Even carbon dioxide, which we all exhale and which is a common component of air, can be lethal in higher concentrations. In 1986, a massive eruption of the volcanic lake Nyos, in Cameroon, Africa, killed people and livestock up to 25 kilometers (about 18 miles) away because it released concentrated CO_2 (Figure 10, see color section). Two years before, a carbon dioxide release from a nearby lake, Monoun, killed 37 people. Occasionally, farmers in the midwestern United States die when they climb into a silo filled with fermenting grain, which releases carbon dioxide.

Nitrogen

Nitrogen is essential to life; it is a key element in proteins. The elemental form contains two nitrogen atoms, written N_2, and is a nontoxic, unreactive gas that makes up 78% of the atmosphere. When pumped into the bloodstream during deep scuba dives, nitrogen gas can cause a euphoria, referred to as nitrogen narcosis, that will be discussed later. Breathing pure nitrogen results in asphyxiation from lack of oxygen, but this is rarely a problem except when a large refrigerated tank of liquid nitrogen breaks in a confined area, displacing oxygen.

A compound of nitrogen, the nitrite anion, is used for curing, preserving, and improving the color of meats—especially bacon. This practice has been controversial, not because nitrite salts are toxic (they are not in modest concentrations), but because, at high temperatures as used in frying, the reaction of nitrite with proteins forms carcinogenic compounds called nitrosamines. The tradeoff (life is filled with tradeoffs!) is that nitrite salts kill dangerous bacteria; thus, nitrites are still added to various meat products despite the fact that cooking the meat can produce carcinogens. In 1987, it was reported that microwaved bacon does not contain much of the cancer-causing nitrosamines, as compared with fried bacon. The difference is the temperature. I prefer the taste of bacon cooked in a microwave oven anyway. This is but one example of a widespread, little-studied phenomenon, the production of toxic agents by cooking food! In that regard, I mention the formation of an acutely toxic aldehyde called acrolein, which is inevitably created when broiling steaks on charcoal or gas grills. Acrolein (which does not contain nitrogen) gives the pleasant, acrid odor to the smoke from a charcoal grill; acrolein is formed from fat striking a very hot surface. Not to worry, your author relishes the occasional charcoal broiled steak.

Another, somewhat bizarre compound of nitrogen is the azide ion. Azide salts are very toxic; neutral azide compounds are also explosive. The only place you will encounter azide salts, such as sodium azide, is in the airbag in your car; these salts are part of the explosive mechanism that deploys the airbag. The disposal of airbags may become a problem because of this compound! Azide ions bind to the active site of the respiratory enzyme cytochrome c oxidase. When this happens, the organism is quickly asphyxiated! Despite this environmental hazard, the next car I buy will have an airbag

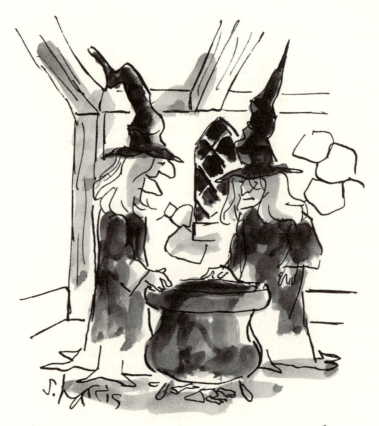

"I DON'T USE IT ANYMORE, SINCE I GOT MY MICROWAVE OVEN."

because I believe there are some risks in life worth taking to obtain other benefits. Beyond their toxic chemical explosive, airbags can also be a physical hazard to infants or small children sitting in the front seat.

Another nitrogen-containing anion known by most people to be toxic is cyanide. The volatile acid form, hydrogen cyanide, is used in gas chambers. The infamous Nazi war criminal, Hermann Goering (and, over the years, several chemists) imbibed cyanide salts to commit suicide. Cyanide, like azide, acts to inhibit the respiratory enzyme. In the southwestern Pacific Ocean, groupers and related fish are stunned by divers who squirt sodium cyanide at them. Although the dose used is not toxic to people or to the fish, it does kill the sensitive corals that create and maintain the reef habitat. Environmentalists should rightly oppose this practice, but few know about it.

Cassava is a staple food for 200 million people in central Africa. This plant, however, contains some cyanide, and if the concentration is high enough, people eating cassava can be poisoned. Young children may die, whereas other people, especially children and women, develop konzo, a disease that irreversibly paralyses their legs. Water can leach cyanide out of cassava, so areas with higher rainfall have less cyanide in their cassava crops. Many people have tasted cyanide when they have bitten into the kernel of an apricot or peach pit, which contains a compound in which cyanide is linked to a sugar. Recall the bitter taste! As I mentioned previously (Chapter 3), this substance, called laetrile, is sold as a nutritional supplement in health food stores and used as a cancer cure in Mexican clinics.

The principal oxides of nitrogen are interesting. First, consider N_2O, nitrous oxide, sometimes referred to as laughing gas. This colorless, odorless gas is still used as an anesthetic in the operating theater and by dental surgeons despite the fact that in rats it is a known teratogen (causes birth defects). Anesthesiologists have no evidence of such an effect in human patients but refrain from using it on pregnant women. Nitrous oxide is occasionally abused by teenagers, who steal tanks of it and use it to become intoxicated. Unfortunately, an overdose can lead to death by asphyxiation.

A closely related compound, nitric oxide (NO) has appeared frequently in the scientific news. Nitric oxide is a nearly colorless, reactive, toxic gas. It reacts with oxygen in the air to form nitrogen dioxide (NO_2), a highly toxic, brown gas. You may have noticed this brown gas at the top of the tall chimneys of plants producing sulfuric acid. The exhaust of automobiles and power plants contains some nitrogen dioxide that is produced by the high-temperature combustion of nitrogen (N_2) from the air. Nitrogen dioxide is toxic because it causes serious lung damage.

Although nitric oxide has a thoroughly bad reputation as a destroyer of atmospheric ozone, a suspected carcinogen, and a precursor of acid rain, your body produces this molecule. Nitric oxide is a naturally generated hormone that has many functions in the body. Nitric oxide is essential to digestion, blood-pressure regulation, antimicrobial defenses, and penile erections. In 1992 the journal *Science* named nitric oxide "molecule of the year" as the importance of NO was becoming understood. In 1998, the Nobel prize in Physiology or Medicine was awarded to Robert F. Furchgott, Louis J. Ignarro, and Ferid Murrad for their discovery of the biological functions of nitric oxide. The nitric oxide formed in the body by enzymes is not altogether good; its derivatives can damage DNA, and it has been implicated in the nerve damage left by strokes.

Some drugs owe their activity to the release of nitric oxide. For example, the highly explosive compound nitroglycerin, tamed by Alfred Nobel in dynamite, has been used for many years to treat heart trouble; Nobel himself used it. Amyl nitrite has been used for years as an illicit sexual stimulant, especially within the gay community; this substance acts to release nitric oxide in the body.

In the body, nitric oxide is produced by an enzyme, nitric oxide synthase (NOS), from the amino acid arginine. Septic shock, a leading cause of death in intensive care wards, seems to result from the body's production of too much nitric oxide. Drugs that inhibit the enzyme NOS are being developed to treat septic shock. In the immune system, nitric oxide can act as a cellular assassin; its mode of action is still under study, but one mechanism has been recognized. A highly destructive ion, peroxynitrite, is formed in the body whenever the superoxide anion, a reactive form of oxygen, encounters nitric oxide. Peroxynitrite is thought to be involved in cancer, in autoimmune inflammations such as arthritis, in heart attacks, and in cell death. Superoxide ion is a toxic byproduct of respiration that is normally controlled by another enzyme, superoxide dismutase. However, when nitric oxide is produced in the presence of free superoxide ion, peroxynitrite is formed at an extremely fast rate, and all hell breaks loose as the saying goes. The neighboring tissue is destroyed by this nasty anion.

Nature is Elemental

The reduced form of nitrogen, ammonia, is familiar to many people in the form of the cleaning agent called household ammonia and in smelling salts. Ammonia is also a huge-commodity chemical manufactured principally as a fertilizer. It is not uncommon for a farmer to have large ammonia tanks (well over 1,000 gallons) to store the very cold, liquefied form of ammonia. Ammonia is injected directly into the soil as a fertilizer (Figure 11, see color section). Of course, farmers are familiar with ammonia in another form—it is a principal constituent of degraded urine; a cow barn reeks of ammonia!

Ammonia was once extensively used as a refrigerant in ice plants and early home refrigerators; this use has been abandoned because the highly volatile ammonia is very toxic if inhaled. Aqueous ammonia is very basic; it will irritate your eyes and can even cause blindness if not washed out. A toxic-gas ordinance in Santa Clara County, California, places very strict limits on the transport and storage of even small tanks of ammonia—despite the fact that no such strict control is exercised for household ammonia, smelling salts, or ammonia fertilizer. Such is the modern, chemophobic world!

An overabundance of ammonia is creating ecological problems. Massive quantities of ammonia are produced by the catalytic reduction of nitrogen from air using hydrogen gas. The worldwide agricultural usage of industrial nitrogen fertilizer to boost crop production has resulted in a glut of reactive nitrogen compounds such as ammonia and nitrates. These nutrients encourage algal blooms that turn clear water into a gooey, green scum. When a thick mat of algae grows, the lowest layer of algae receives no light and dies. The decomposition of dead algae uses up the oxygen in the water, and as a result, fish and shellfish die off. Elsewhere, I note that excess ammonia also promotes the upsurge in dangerous toxic algae called red tides. Part of the problem is that much agricultural nitrogen is not used efficiently and leaches into waterways.

The combination of household ammonia with laundry bleach or the bleach in some scouring powders represents a little-recognized danger. A rapid reaction of bleach with ammonia produces a toxic gas, chloramine, and eventually a soluble toxic chemical, hydrazine. These common household chemicals are also toxic individually and should be kept away from children. Together, they have the potential to kill adults.

Phosphorus

In various forms, phosphorus is required for life. The biologically active form of phosphorus is the phosphate ion. Phosphates are present in many biological compounds such as phospholipids, DNA, and the energy-storage molecule, ATP. Some synthetic phosphorus derivatives can be very toxic. One example is white phosphorus; this elemental form is toxic even if it just comes in contact with your skin. White phosphorus has been used as a component of incendiary bombs.

Because phosphorus is so easily transformed by oxygen, only phosphate derivatives are found in nature. High levels of phosphate salts that serve as fertilizers can cause environmental problems by stimulating the growth of algae, as described above (Figure 12, see color section). Such overgrowth of algae in a body of water is called eutrophication.

A toxic, synthetic compound of phosphorus is found in match heads—these should be kept away from small children.

Arsenic

Arsenic lies below phosphorus in the periodic table. From reading fictional stories such as *Arsenic and Old Lace,* most people know that arsenic is poisonous. Its action is caused by the arsenate ion substituting for the structurally similar phosphate ion in biological compounds, thereby interfering with vital, biochemical transformations. For many years, its toxicity was unrecognized; arsenic was used as a pesticide in agriculture, and Swiss mountain climbers once consumed arsenic in the belief that it gave them strength. Long ago, it was used to treat tuberculosis. Because some arsenic is present in shellfish, arsenic got an undeserved reputation as an aphrodisiac. The amount of arsenic in mussels can exceed that allowed in drinking water. Other shellfish, including shrimp, also contain arsenic, but the arsenic in these shellfish is in a form that is not metabolized and thought not to be a health hazard. Because the general public is unaware that arsenic resides in some of their favorite foods, there is no misplaced public health concern.

There are claims that arsenic in tiny quantities may be an essential nutrient for humans. Up to 12 micrograms per day may be healthful; this is such a tiny amount that you could not see it without a microscope. If these claims are true, the mechanism of action is un-

Nature is Elemental

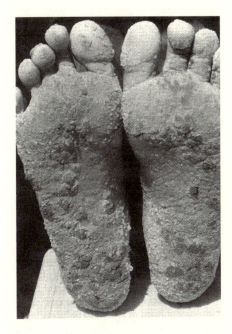

Figure 13. One symptom
of arsenic poisoning.

known, but there is evidence that human populations may differ
sharply in how they metabolize arsenic. For example, there is a
group of indigenous villagers in Chile who, for many generations, apparently have been drinking water laced with dangerous levels of arsenic, but who have no signs of cancer. For most people, however, as
little as one-tenth of a gram of arsenic can be lethal in some forms
such as arsenate. Other chemical forms of arsenic are also quite toxic.
Arsenic poisoning is cumulative; tiny amounts of arsenic from tap
water build up in the bodies of victims over many years, until physical symptoms emerge, as illustrated in Figure 13. Some evidence
points toward a threshold concentration below which the body can
excrete arsenic by converting it to nontoxic forms. There is an anecdotal report that hops extract arsenic from the soil in which they
grow and that beer, which is brewed from hops, may contain traces
of arsenic.

India has a health crisis in West Bengal, where high levels of arsenic have leached into thousands of village wells. An estimated
200,000 people already have arsenic-induced skin lesions; some also
have hardened patches of skin that may develop into cancer. This

problem started with drilling deeper wells, which were needed to grow the new, irrigation-intensive rice crops associated with the Green Revolution.

A similar problem is faced in Bangladesh, where tube wells were sunk into the ground to reach the water table, which unfortunately contains arsenic deposits. Arsenic contamination of drinking water has been declared by Allan H. Smith, an epidemiologist at the University of California, Berkeley, to be "the highest cancer risk ever found." Tragically, the organization UNICEF was the main proponent of digging these wells, but its intentions were to solve a different health problem. The use of these wells did lower the mortality rates attributed to cholera and diarrhea, the nation's major killers, whose cause stemmed from drinking water taken from hand-dug wells or natural ponds shared by bathing cows. Solving one problem seems to have created a worse one.

In 2000, the US Environmental Protection Agency (EPA) proposed lowering the limit on arsenic levels allowed in drinking water from 50 parts per billion to 5 parts per billion. An environmental group proposed a limit of 3 parts per billion, the lowest amount considered feasible with current technology. Attaining the standard proposed by the EPA is estimated to cost between $28 and $85 a year per household, depending on the size of the community. Communities in the Southwest would be the most affected. For example, Albuquerque, New Mexico, had an arsenic level of 14 parts per billion and Norman, Oklahoma, had a level of 36 parts per billion. The proposed EPA limit would provide a cancer risk of 1 in 10,000; most of these cancers are treatable. This proposal was prompted by studies of skin cancer in Taiwan that may be linked to arsenic in drinking water.

Oxygen

The elemental form of oxygen, a diatomic molecule, is required for aerobic life, but in high concentrations, oxygen gas, O_2, is very toxic. Pure oxygen at a pressure of 1.5 to 1.7 atmospheres, which equals 21–24 pounds per square inch, can cause convulsions, brain damage, and death. This effect is discussed later as a problem in deep scuba diving.

Another chemical form of oxygen that is much in the news is ozone. Ozone, the triatomic form of oxygen, is quite toxic in fairly low concentrations. Since the early 1900s, ozone has been used to disinfect water supplies in France. Ozone spontaneously decomposes, and therefore its activity is quickly lost as water flows through the delivery system. Ozone has an acrid odor, which you may have smelled just after an electrical short (or a lightning flash), which produces ozone. Perhaps you have smelled ozone in an electric street car.

Ozone is a well-publicized air pollutant. It is produced by the interaction of sunlight with nitrogen oxides in the formation of smog. Ozone is very reactive; it attacks and cleaves (breaks apart) carbon–carbon double bonds. The long carbon chains in natural and most synthetic rubber contain such double bonds. That is why wetsuits and rubber tires are more rapidly degraded in Los Angeles, where the smoggy atmosphere contains higher concentrations of ozone than in other areas. Of course, the tissue in your lungs is also easily damaged by ozone.

Several years ago, there was an ozone problem associated with the high-flying Boeing 747-S, a long-range aircraft that can fly nonstop for distances equal to Tokyo to New York. At very high altitudes and particular latitudes where atmospheric ozone is more concentrated, dangerous levels of ozone from outside the aircraft were being introduced into the passenger compartment. Flight attendants and some passengers became ill from the dangerously high ozone levels. This problem has since been solved by taking advantage of the fact that ozone is intrinsically unstable—it tends to decompose spontaneously into ordinary oxygen. The first solution to this ozone contamination involved heating the intake air to induce the transformation of ozone into oxygen. The result was a hot, uncomfortable airplane flight. Later, a catalyst, probably containing platinum, was used to promote this reaction at lower temperatures.

In the 1940s, some movie theaters in Oregon and the San Francisco Bay Area installed ozone generators in their restrooms—they even advertised this! The effect was to reduce odors (more specifically the movie-goers ability to detect odors). Fortunately, most customers spent little time in these toxic rooms!

In the 1990s, I read a surprising advertisement for a household ozone generator that was said to "clean the air Nature's own way." I doubt it! First, recall that ozone has a disagreeable odor, so any product that generated it would have few sales, indeed. Furthermore, the well-known toxicity of ozone would lead some consumers to file lawsuits if ozone were actually being generated. Nevertheless, this

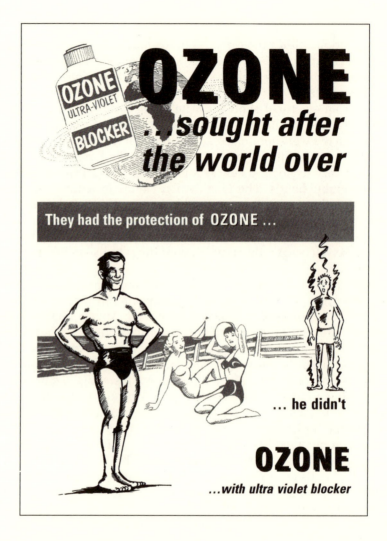

company was taking advantage of the public's scientific innocence to sell a bogus product. Apparently, one cannot successfully sue over simple scientific fraud!

You may be surprised to learn that, in other places, ozone is a "good guy." In the upper atmosphere, ultraviolet light creates a thin ozone layer that absorbs damaging ultraviolet radiation, thereby lowering the incidence of skin cancer and plant damage on the surface of the Earth. The problem of the ozone hole is discussed later.

Sulfur

Oxygen's relative, sulfur, is highly toxic in the form of hydrogen sulfide, H_2S. This analog of water is a foul-smelling gas that has an odor like rotten eggs; after a short exposure, however, your nose quickly loses its ability to detect hydrogen sulfide. Hydrogen sulfide is nearly as toxic as hydrogen cyanide, although initially we can smell H_2S at much lower concentrations. Trace amounts of this noxious gas probably account for the foul smell in automobile exhaust—from the actions of the catalytic converter.

Another common chemical derived from sulfur, sulfur dioxide, is a corrosive pollutant and is discussed later as a precursor of acid rain. Sulfur dioxide is formed by the burning of sulfur-rich coal and oil. It is also used in winemaking to kill wild yeasts, which cause unwanted fermentation products, and to prevent spoilage by reaction of the wine with oxygen in the air. California wines containing sulfites are labeled as such. If a wine contains more than 10 ppm sulfite, it must be so marked. The legally allowed upper limit is 350 ppm. Sulfites also keep foods from spoiling and thus are used as preservatives in a huge variety of foods and beverages. Some individuals, about 1% of the population, are quite allergic to sulfur dioxide and its water-soluble derivative, the sulfite ion. Up to 5% of asthmatics are sulfite-sensitive. To protect those with sulfite sensitivity, the FDA prohibits sulfite use in salad bars and requires food containing sulfites to be labeled as such.

Selenium

Because it is just below sulfur in the periodic table, selenium can be thought of as sulfur's big brother. Like sulfur, selenium is essential for life—but only in trace quantities. Insufficient selenium results in degenerative muscle disease. Selenium is also thought by some to protect against cancer. A recent double-blind study of 600 people who took selenium supplements over a 10-year-period showed that they developed 71% fewer prostate cancers, 67% fewer esophageal cancers, 62% fewer colorectal cancers, and 46% fewer lung cancers than did a comparable group of 600 people who took placebo tablets. The daily dose in this study, 200 micrograms of selenium, was three times the presently recommended level. The main dietary sources of selenium are meats, poultry, fish, cereals, and vegetables such as mushrooms and asparagus. Brazil nuts in their shell are loaded with selenium; two nuts a day provide more than the daily requirement. Ingesting the form of selenium in foods may be more efficacious than that from supplements, because the selenium is probably present in the foods as a naturally occurring amino acid. Selenium's beneficial effects are thought to arise from its role as an antioxidant. People with low levels of selenium in their blood are three times more likely to die of a heart attack; selenium raises blood levels of HDL, the good cholesterol.

Now for the bad news: in larger amounts, elemental selenium and most of its compounds are quite toxic. Supplemental doses of selenium above 750 micrograms daily can be toxic. In 1984, an accidental excess of 125 times the recommended amount of selenium was present in some health supplements that are thought to have caused 11 deaths. Symptoms of selenium overdoses include loss of hair and fingernails, nausea, vomiting, and fatigue. Higher incidences of liver and stomach cancers, Hodgkin's disease, and leukemia are also associated with ingestion of excess selenium. Selenium accumulates in water and concentrates by evaporation in some drainage pits in the Central Valley of California. There, it is ingested by waterfowl, some of which die as a result of selenium poisoning. Early in the 19th century, thousands of cattle, horses, and sheep in Wyoming, Utah, Nebraska, and South Dakota died from ingesting grasses and grains loaded with this element, which is in overabundance in the soils of many areas west of the Mississippi River. Clearly, selenium is a classic example of something for which a little is essential and too much is deadly.

The compound selenium sulfide is a common ingredient in shampoos and topical ointments for eczema and dandruff; be careful not to imbibe any of this substance. The gas hydrogen selenide (to which we are not exposed) has an even more noxious odor and is even more poisonous than its cousin, hydrogen sulfide.

Fluorine

A family of elements called halogens is located in a vertical column on the right side of the periodic table. The lightest element in the halogen family, fluorine, is very unusual. The violently reactive elemental form, fluorine gas, does not occur in nature. Only specialists encounter elemental fluorine. On the other hand, the fluoride anion is often in the news; for several decades, small amounts of fluoride salts have been added to the water supplies of most municipalities in the United States (from 0.7 to 1.2 parts of fluoride per million parts of water). For adults and children alike, the dental benefits from using fluoridated water, such as reduction of cavities, are widely accepted, despite continued opposition that claims this public-health measure is actually a public-health hazard. It is true that, at about 80-fold higher concentrations, fluoride increases the incidence of some cancers. Danish mineral workers exposed to very high levels of fluoride have a suspiciously high incidence of bladder cancers. This is a classic case of a dose-response mechanism at work; again, the *amount* of the substance determines its relative safety, not just the presence or absence of it.

Fluoride, in the form of sodium fluoride, is added in small amounts (0.15%) to toothpaste with a warning for children not to ingest this substance. At present, 155 million Americans, or 62% of the population, live in places where the water is fluoridated. Most people also use fluoride toothpaste. Because of this increased exposure to fluoride and a better diet, Americans' dental health has greatly improved in recent decades. Many homes, however, have filtration systems that remove fluoride from the water. Many homeowners do not recognize this downside of their water-filtration units.

In contrast to the United States, Britain remains stubbornly resistant to the fluoridation of water. Only 10% of the British population, or about 5.5 million people, live in places where the water is fluoridated. People living in regions with fluoridated water have fewer cavities than the average population, which is not drinking fluoridated water.

A curious fact about fluoride concerns the use of bottled water. The extensive consumption of bottled water is at an all-time high—on average, 12.7 gallons per person was consumed in the United States in 1998. Some dentists worry that bottled water contains little fluoride and therefore its heavy use deprives children of the benefits of fluoride in the water supply.

Teas, both herbal and regular, contain considerable amounts of fluoride—some are reported to be above the levels used in fluoridation. For example, Twinings Earl Grey Tea contains 2.07 parts per million; Lipton's English Breakfast Tea, 2.17 ppm; and Nestea Instant Tea, 7.58 ppm. Many individuals opposed to fluoridation drink tea without realizing that it contains fluoride.

An acid derivative of fluorine, hydrofluoric acid, is very toxic, even at low concentrations. It can penetrate the skin, causing degeneration of connective tissues. The treatment for this malady is quite painful: injection of calcium salts directly into the affected area. Perhaps you have heard of the characteristic that hydrofluoric acid can "eat through" glass; that is why it is used to make frosted light-bulbs. Oil refineries, even in some metropolitan areas, use large quantities of hydrofluoric acid and a related substance, boron trifluoride, as catalysts to convert petroleum fractions into high-octane gasoline. Hydrofluoric acid is sometimes shipped by rail, in tank-car quantities. I regard this a dangerous practice; to me, the risk is not worth the benefit. This is one example of a real hazard not recognized by the general public, in contrast to some hypothetical hazards that monopolize the news.

Organofluorine compounds are exceedingly rare in nature. The carbon–fluorine bond is very stable and therefore is usually unreactive. One organofluorine compound, the polymer Teflon, is biologically inert. Fluorine atoms have been introduced into several pharmaceutical agents. For example, Ultravate (halobetasol propionate) is a topical ointment that is more efficacious than the naturally occurring hydrocortisone. Fluorinated drugs retain their potency longer in the body because they are more difficult to degrade. A small fluorinated molecule, halothane, was introduced as a general anesthetic in 1956; its low toxicity, low flammability, and high stability have kept halothane as a dominant anesthetic today.

The chlorofluorocarbons (CFCs) were introduced in 1931 as refrigerants and have also been used as aerosol propellants. Their use is now being phased out. This change is not because the CFCs are toxic—they are not—but because they are decomposed in the upper atmosphere by intense ultraviolet radiation to form chlorine radicals (Cl•) that catalyze the destruction of ozone, creating the ozone hole, a topic discussed further on. Thus, these stable substances are indirectly hazardous.

A very toxic fluorocarbon, fluoroacetic acid, is used as a rat poison (in the form of its sodium salt). Mistakenly recognizing this substance as the naturally occurring salt of vinegar, the acetate ion, enzymes take up this toxic imposter and are caused to "commit suicide."

Chlorine

The element chlorine is the environmentalist's Public Enemy Number One. Why is that, and is it justified? This is a complex, still-evolving issue. The elemental form of chlorine is very reactive—it was used as a poison gas in World War I. Today, chlorine gas and its neutralized cousin, hypochlorite ion, which is used in bleaches such as Chlorox, are added to swimming pools. Chlorine is introduced into most municipal water supplies to kill bacteria and other hazardous biological agents. The practice of disinfecting water by the addition of chlorine is being questioned because small amounts of chloroform are formed during the purification of water. Chloroform was once used in some toothpastes (5%, or five parts per hundred), in certain throat lozenges, and in some cough syrups (up to 15%). Little or no evidence suggests that these practices resulted in a health hazard. In 1995, the EPA suggested that drinking water in the United States should contain no more than 0.004 parts per million of chloroform. They selected this limit for humans by extrapolating data taken from studies of high-level chlorine exposure to animals. Mice developed liver tumors after exposure to massive daily doses of chloroform pumped into their stomachs over several months! Many scientists have recently called for more realistic studies that take into account the concentrations of toxic chemicals and mechanisms by which they affect cells.

The principal controversy involving chlorine is over dioxin, a general term given to several chlorinated compounds. The toxicity of dioxins shows tremendous variation depending on the animal species that is used for the test. Initial studies with guinea pigs indicated that 6×10^{-6} g of dioxin killed 50% of these test animals; later studies with hamsters showed dioxin to be *1,000 times less toxic.* Conversely, lake trout fry are very sensitive to dioxin. At concentrations of just 60 parts per trillion, dioxin kills 50% of the fry.

The initial, alarming studies on guinea pigs suggested that dioxin is the most toxic industrial chemical known. This conclusion led to drastic action. For example, in 1983, the US government bought up and evacuated an entire town, Times Beach, Missouri, because dioxin was found in the soil. Dioxin also was found as a contaminant in Agent Orange and in the chemical sludge of the infamous Love Canal.

A more realistic view of the toxicity of dioxin toward humans came from an incident in Italy. In 1976, a huge industrial accident occurred in Seveso, Italy, spilling very large amounts of dioxin over the town and surrounding countryside. Subsequent analysis showed that large amounts of dioxin remained in the bodies of the residents, but the effect was by no means lethal. After nearly 20 years, skin rashes (chloracne) and some other ailments have been attributed to this exposure to dioxin. However, an epidemiological study of workers in a US chemical plant who had been exposed to high levels of dioxin for more than a year revealed a 46% higher cancer rate than in the general public. According to the American Cancer Society, four out of ten people will experience cancer in their lifetimes; two out of ten will die of cancer. Although dioxin is clearly a human carcinogen, it is not nearly as deadly as the original claim.

How do dioxins exert their effect? Every cell in the body has a protein receptor which binds flat molecules. This "Ah receptor," acting like a lock, binds dioxins, which serve as a key and accelerate normal development, impair infertility, and cause diseases, perhaps including cancer. Although other pollutants can also turn on this Ah receptor, dioxins fit the receptor best and are therefore very potent toxins. The Ah receptor is thought to have a use in normal development, but its natural function is presently unknown.

A more recent Environmental Protection Agency (EPA) study of the dioxin problem came out in 1995 and was the source of intense controversy. The environmental-action organization Greenpeace and its allies have been accused of overly influencing the EPA regarding dioxin. Principally because of the dioxin controversy, some scientists are worried that the EPA might curtail or ban the production of chlorine and compounds containing chlorine. The fears that chlorine-containing compounds may imitate the effects of estrogen and cause male infertility and female breast cancer add to this issue. The media have given an unbalanced treatment of this complicated topic, and it remains unresolved.

Why not just ban the production of dioxins? The problem is much more complex. Incineration of municipal waste produces dioxins and related toxic chlorinated compounds. This is the major reason that environmentalists are opposed to incineration of wastes— no matter how modern the facility or where the incinerator is located. In fact, rural households that burn their garbage in barrels out back may be producing the most dioxin. A handful of such fires can spew out as much dioxin as a large municipal incinerator. Steel mills, metal smelters, and motor vehicles burning unleaded fuels also produce large amounts of toxic equivalents.

Some of the worst cases of contamination by dioxins and the chlorinated insecticide DDT are found in the Arctic, thousands of miles away from any industrial center. These environmental pollutants are a health threat to whales and dolphins, which store large amounts of these oil-soluble compounds in their body fat.

There is an ongoing debate as to the proportion of these chlorinated compounds produced by humans, called anthropogenic production, versus the proportion found in nature. For example, dioxins and similar compounds are produced by natural forest fires. There are 200,000 such fires per year worldwide, caused largely by lightning. Estimates are that Canada alone produces 130 pounds of dioxins each year in this way. Dioxins are also known to be generated in fresh, uncontaminated garden compost piles and in municipal sewage sludge—presumably by natural enzymes acting on organic matter, all of which contain some chloride. These chlorinated toxins are not new. Dioxin and other organochlorine compounds have been found in ancient sediments, dating back 8,000 years. Moreover, large concentrations of dioxins have been discovered in ancient, pristine lake sediments in Mississippi. There are 2,400 known, naturally occurring organochlorine compounds, and the natural global depository of all such substances is estimated to be 6 billion tons! Most of these compounds are thought to have a natural origin. Another related chemical containing bromine illustrates this dilemma. A brominated phenol, 2,4,6-tribromophenol, designated by the EPA as a hazardous waste, is produced naturally in substantial amounts by several species of marine acorn worms.

Seawater contains 26×10^{15} tons of chloride (19 g of chloride per liter of seawater). Chloride is present in every cell of every living organism; hydrogen chloride is in each of our stomachs. Myeloperoxidase, an enzyme in our white blood cells, generates hypochlorite ion in cellular regions in the course of an immune response against infection. This mechanism may be involved in promoting atherosclerosis by solidifying low-density lipoprotein (LDL), the "bad" cholesterol. This controversy represents a natural risk–benefit situation that is out of our control.

A total ban on chlorine products has been compared to an attempt to repeal the law of gravity. This element is essential to life and to safeguarding our health. The most prudent course for public policy is to identify the nature, concentrations, and origins of the most toxic organochlorine compounds in a balanced risk assessment. For instance, we need to remember the number of lives saved by disinfecting water with chlorine. When chlorination of the water supply was interrupted in Peru, a serious outbreak of cholera followed. Estimates are that 25,000 children in less-developed countries die each year of waterborne diseases.

Iodine

Another halogen, iodine, is required for life; your body makes an iodinated compound in the thyroid, which is why table salt contains

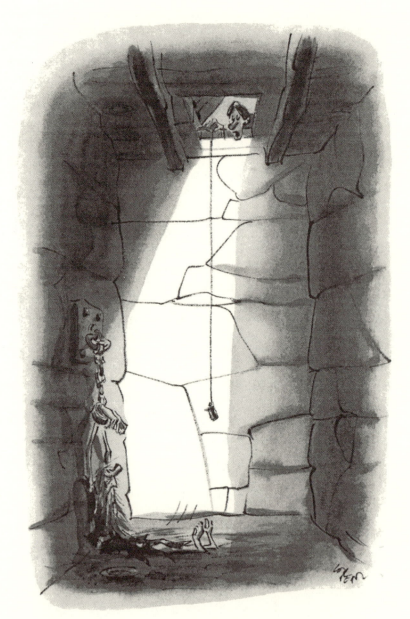

"No cause for alarm—we're checking for radon emissions."

added iodide. An excess of this iodinated thyroid hormone is toxic; for this reason, thyroid glands from beef have been declared unfit for human consumption. Elemental iodine is a mild disinfectant and is sometimes used to purify water on camping trips, although it imparts an unpleasant flavor to the treated water. Not surprisingly, excess iodine is not good for you. On the other hand, if a population consumes heavily refined salt, which is stripped of its natural iodine, many individuals become ill. This lack of iodine has been estimated to have resulted in 10 million cases of mental retardation in China. Iodine is yet another example that a small amount of something is necessary but more can be dangerous.

Radon

An inert gas is deadly? One of the so-called inert gases, radon, is much in the news. Some people are renovating their homes to remove small amounts of radon from their basements; others are abandoning their wells because the water contains traces of radon. In some states, before a property can be sold, it must be made free from radon. The problem stems from the fact that radon is a mildly radioactive decay product of uranium, which is found in many parts of the Earth's crust. Radon can seep out of rocks and become trapped inside houses. Over a long period of time, residents could be exposed to possibly dangerous doses of gamma radiation from radon. Based on high lung cancer rates among uranium miners, it was calculated that up to 10% of all lung cancers in some countries might be caused by radon. A National Research Council study estimates that radon contributes to about 12% of all lung cancer deaths each year in the United States—between 15,000 and 22,000. Almost 90% of these victims were smokers. Thus, eliminating the deadly combination of smoking and radon exposure would prevent almost all such lung cancer deaths.

In 1996, an epidemiologic study in Finland challenged radon's deadly reputation. This study compared radon levels in the homes of 1,000 people with lung cancer with those of more than 1,000 people without cancer. Radon exposure did not seem to increase cancer risk. This study raises doubts about the risks associated with low doses in the home, even though there is little question that radon exposure can cause lung cancer among smokers. The uncertainty about the danger of radon also concerns the dose level. I return to this issue in Chapter 10, which discusses ionizing radiation.

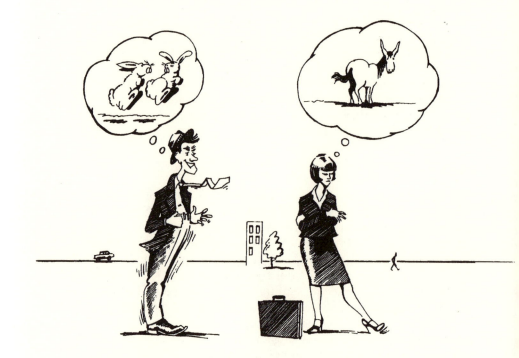

"sophisticated signalling"

7

Natural and Unnatural Molecules in the Environment

THERE ARE MANY NATURAL substances that can strongly influence our lives. Some are hazardous; others are necessary or useful. I begin by describing some toxic natural substances.

Perilous Natural Toxins

Domoic acid, a toxin produced by a common West Coast marine algae, is taken up by shellfish such as mussels. When people consume these mussels, they are poisoned. Ingestion of domoic acid overstimulates and destroys nerve cells. Victims lose their memory; they cannot tell you what they had for breakfast! Domoic acid poisoning of a bird population has been blamed for the 1961 "crazed seabird invasion" of Capitola, California, that inspired Alfred Hitchcock's movie, *The Birds.* Earlier, I mentioned some other marine organisms which produce dangerous toxins, such as those involved in red tides.

A more infamous toxin is known as fugu poison. Fugu are puffer fish, which are a Japanese delicacy. The polar, spheroid tetrodotoxin molecule is extremely toxic because it blocks the sodium channels in nerve cells. The effects of tetrodotoxin are described in ancient literature. Hieroglyphics of several fifth-dynasty Egyptian tombs (about 2700 B.C.) depict a poisonous puffer fish. In the same period, Chinese writing warned of eating certain types of puffer fish found around the China coast. Tetrodotoxin is concentrated in the liver and ovaries of

155

these fish. Specially trained chefs in Japan prepare puffer fish so that these poisonous organs are removed; occasionally, they make a mistake—that produces the excitement associated with eating fugu. (I have always turned down this dish when it was offered.) Tetrodotoxin is 10 times more toxic than black widow spider venom and more than 10,000 times as deadly as cyanide. However, some related substances such as palytoxin from sea organisms have toxicities nearly 100 times that of tetrodotoxin. Surprisingly, puffer fish raised in laboratory environments are not poisonous. Seemingly, the toxin is introduced by an as-yet-unidentified microorganism.

A similar substance, batrachotoxin, which inactivates muscles, is secreted by poisonous green and black frogs in Colombia. One of the deadliest natural substances known, the batrachotoxin contained in a one-inch frog could kill 100 people! Natives in Columbia use this frog skin to prepare blow-gun dart points for hunting. The frogs also seem to obtain this toxin from something in their environment. When raised in captivity, they are also not toxic.

Nature's most poisonous predators—creatures like tarantulas, scorpions, rattlesnakes, and Gila monsters—use their own natural hypodermic needles (scorpion stingers and snake fangs, for example) to inject poisonous venoms into their prey. These venoms contain many different chemicals but the most toxic agents are peptides, small proteinlike molecules. To be effective, these toxins must be injected directly into the muscle because digestive enzymes in the stomach would degrade and inactivate them in the same way that proteins in food are digested. For this reason, in an emergency, a companion can safely come to the aid of a snakebite victim by sucking the venom out of an incision around the puncture wound. Ingesting a small amount of venom seemingly does no serious harm to the "good Samaritan." Venoms from these poisonous animals contain other peptides that can be used as medicines. With the advent of DNA engineering, almost any peptide can be manufactured, so that these venoms provide new hunting grounds for the development of new medicines. These drugs cannot be given orally but instead must be injected into the muscle to avoid being deactivated in the digestive tract. New treatments for diabetes, heart failure, blood clots, and brain disorders are being derived from substances found in natural toxic venoms.

A native plant soon causes newcomers to California to learn to watch themselves, their children, and their dogs while walking in the coastal forests. Firefighters already know the danger in the leaves, roots, and stems of the plant called poison oak. The active ingredient in poison oak is urushiol, a general term for phenolic compounds that contain side chains 17 carbons long. These oily side chains help this poisonous substance penetrate the skin and remain there until a delayed allergic reaction takes place. Even an amount that would fit on a pinhead is sufficient to cause rashes in 500 sensitive people. Forest-fire fighters are greatly endangered by burning poison oak because the active agent may be carried in ash and dust particles in smoke from burning foliage and cause damage in their lungs as well as skin rashes.

Aphrodisiacs

From antiquity, human societies have searched for drugs to enhance sexual activity and desire. Such potents are called aphrodisiacs after Aphrodite, the Greek goddess of love and beauty. Today, some pharmaceutical companies have research programs to discover agents to treat impotence in human males. A male potency drug, Viagra, or sildenafil citrate, manufactured by Pfizer was approved by the FDA in 1998. Strictly speaking, Viagra is not an aphrodisiac because it does not stimulate arousal. However, this drug sustains erections, and therefore many people consider it an aphrodisiac.

What about the ancient sexual remedies? Did any of these natural substances really work? Do they have a scientific basis, or were they just placebos? Are these substances dangerous? The answers to all these questions are a qualified yes. Let's examine a few celebrated cases.

Corynanthe yohimbine, an Asian and Middle Eastern plant, was commonly used for its sexually stimulating properties over a thousand years ago. The active agent, yohimbine, has long been used as a sexual stimulant for domestic animals and recently with some success to treat erectile impotency in human males. The use of yohimbine by the ancients had some merit; however, its side effects include rapid heartbeat and high blood pressure.

Spanish fly (cantharides), an extremely toxic, powerful irritant to the blood vessels, was commonly used as an aphrodisiac during the Middle Ages in both Europe and China. This powder was extracted from a variety of dried blister beetles. The infamous Marquis de Sade

Natural and Unnatural Molecules in the Environment

gave some of this potion to several prostitutes; a few of them died! One such agent, mylabris, is still used in China today as an aphrodisiac and to induce abortions.

A revered ancient aphrodisiac was derived from the purple root of the Asian mandrake plant (*Mandrigora officinarum*). Its use as a sexual stimulant is described in the Bible (Genesis 30:14–17), by the Roman naturalist Pliny (23–79 A.D.), and by Dioscorides, a 1st-century Greek pharmacist. Extracts of the mandrake plant are known to have sedative and narcotic properties, which could explain its use as a sexual agent.

Modern quests for new aphrodisiacs have focused on medicines with neurotransmitter action. For example, the neurotransmitter dopamine stimulates sexual activity. A side effect of L-dopa, a medicine used to treat Parkinson's disease that raises dopamine levels, is increased sexual arousal in 4 out of 7 male patients. Serotonin is another neurotransmitter known to modulate sexual behavior. Several drugs known to raise serotonin levels by inhibiting the re-uptake of serotonin have reportedly increased libido in both male and female patients. Several of these drugs have side effects such as drowsiness and headaches. With the possible exception of Viagra, there are still no safe or reliable aphrodisiacs, but it is only a matter of time until such drugs are discovered because of the large potential market and increased understanding of brain chemistry.

Another approach to developing sexually stimulating drugs is to enhance the production of the hormone NO (nitric oxide), which is known to stimulate penile erection. However, this gaseous hormone (discussed in Chapter 6) has many effects in various parts of the body, so dangerous side effects might accompany any such drug. Homosexuals have employed an illicit drug, referred to as "poppers," which releases NO. Combining Viagra and poppers is very dangerous and can be lethal.

Pheromones

One of the most interesting physiological detections of molecules is the phenomenon related to pheromones. A pheromone is a substance produced by an organism that elicits a specific response in another

Natural and Unnatural Molecules in the Environment

member of the same species. The response to a pheromone is "hard-wired" (inborn) in each species. Pheromones are secreted externally to regulate the organism's external environment by influencing others of its own kind. They are best known in the insect world; insects use pheromones as trail markers, sex attractants, and alarm signals, and for many other activities. The sensitivity to these substances is such that a few hundred molecules of pheromone per cubic centimeter can elicit a response! The gypsy moth attractant, gyplure, has been isolated (20 milligrams from 500,000 gypsy moths), identified by chemical analysis, and synthesized by organic chemists. This attractant has been used in bait traps to eradicate these destructive moths, which have denuded millions of acres of pine forests in the northeastern United States. Scientists have tricked male gypsy moths into copulating with filter paper, just by dousing it with the sublime female gypsy moth scent.

Similarly, the sex pheromones of silkworm moths, American cockroaches, and queen honeybees have been identified and reproduced in the laboratory. In an interesting application, you can intercept an ant trail by neutralizing the ant's acid pheromone (formic acid) with a base—a paste of baking soda will do. Pheromones are also involved in the following response: when a bee or wasp stings, their angry brethren come to sting at the same spot, an attack that is directed from afar by alarm and marker pheromones. Beekeepers who have been stung, even once, are careful to wash the garment they wore at the time, to remove the marker pheromone.

Bacteria also have been found to emit pheromones that ward off predators and cause related bacteria to gather. This subject is in its infancy but may have medical applications.

Higher animals also have pheromones. For example, civetone from the civet cat and muskone from the musk deer are known sex pheromones. These unusual cyclic compounds have been synthesized and are used as perfume bases for humans. Do humans have pheromones? It seems so, but the evidence is scanty. The striking sexual differences in the ability of humans to smell certain substances is based on indirect evidence. Consider, for example, exaltolide. This unnatural substance is detected by sexually mature women most strongly at the time of ovulation but not by young girls or men. If a man has been injected with the female sex hormone estrogen, however, he is able to smell exaltolide! It was also found that the abilities of human subjects to smell exaltolide paralleled their abilities to detect certain steroid hormones.

Natural and Unnatural Molecules in the Environment

Most animals are attractive to the opposite sex only when receptive to mating. For example, male dogs come from a considerable distance when a bitch is in heat—a pheromone is responsible for this attraction. But can people detect and distinguish other people this way? Humans are said not to dislike their own body odors (of all types) but typically dislike the odors of others—especially the odors of the opposite sex. If you believe the deodorant advertisements, women seem to be more strongly repelled by male odors than vice versa.

Excessive bathing and perfumery may have suppressed these ancient, unused avenues of interaction in humans. Sex and odor are intertwined in obscure ways. Recall that Napoleon wrote Josephine, "Not to wash, I will soon be home." Pheromones are thought to affect behavior at subconscious levels. Can chemical signals from one human be detected by another without being consciously experienced as an odor? As you will see below, commercial perfume makers are now employing what they believe to be human pheromones.

Perhaps the best evidence for the existence of human pheromones involves menstrual synchrony. When women live together in close quarters for months at a time, their menstrual cycles begin to coincide. This phenomenon has been studied carefully and traced to unidentified odors in underarm sweat. Other studies have shown that a mother can identify the odor of her newborn infant or older child by smelling a t-shirt worn previously by her child, correctly discriminating it from a shirt worn by another child of the same age. Further, infants prefer breast pads from their own mothers over pads from other mothers.

Pheromones have sometimes elicited their effects between species. Consider the following example. The pungent, aromatic French truffle is a fungus used in foie gras, pates, and omelets. This gourmet delight is literally worth its weight in gold. The ancient Babylonians are believed to be the first people to have observed wild pigs digging up this underground fungus. Today, pigs and dogs are still used to harvest truffles. Whereas pigs have the better sense of smell, dogs are less inclined to gobble up the valuable fungus. Pigs can locate truffles growing as deep as 1 meter underground. Recently, it was discovered that the attractive substance in truffles is from a steroid, 5α-androst-16-en-3α-ol. This compound, which has a very peculiar musk odor, is a pheromone that is also given off by boars during their premating behavior. It is fascinating that truffles secrete traces of this same steroidal pheromone. It is unclear why a fungus and a mammal would both use the same chemical. Men also secrete this compound in their underarm sweat, and this substance is also found in the urine of women. Is this steroid also a human pheromone? No one is absolutely certain, but the presence of this molecule does appear to make men more attentive to women. It is interesting that about half the human population can detect the odor of this molecule; of these, half intensely dislike the odor, and the other half find it somewhat pleasant. There is an alcohol group in this pheromone, and when it is moved to the opposite side of the steroid molecule, an isomer called 3-ß-ol is formed. This beta isomer is a female hormone attractive to men (and to boars). Thus, pigs and humans seem to share a common pheromone.

A perfume maker has introduced both male and female perfumes containing the two isomeric steroids discussed above. These steroid pheromones are sometimes blended with a derivative called androstenone, which is claimed to be the essence of aggression in males. For example, it is reported that men in the violent wing of a prison are high secretors of this molecule.

Mixtures of these apparent human pheromones are advertised on the internet. They have many claimed uses. It is said that some furniture companies have used these substances in their showrooms and that such pheromones influence where men and women customers sit, depending on the particular steroid! A perfume called desire 22 contains a pheromone product claimed to sexually attract men. These steroid pheromones are very expensive per unit weight, but they are apparently effective in tiny concentrations. Androstenone costs about $8,000 per gram!

Some pheromones are not especially volatile; at room temperature, very few of these steroid molecules would be in the gas phase, and they may have no detectable odor. On the other hand, as you have seen, there is a lot of circumstantial evidence suggesting that steroid molecules similar to cholesterol have sex-specific effects on animals, including humans. By spraying human androstenes on seats in a theater, women become more likely and men less likely to sit on those seats. How do humans detect these apparently odorless molecules? Our bodies have a tiny structure known as the vomeronasal organ (VNO) that is speculated to carry chemical messages to the brain, but may not elicit the sensation of smell or odor. Previously, the VNO was considered an inactive vestige of our evolutionary past, even though it was known to be active in some mammals. Perhaps the VNO in humans detects pheromones?

Man-Made Chemicals in the Environment

Insecticides

Most insecticides were originally added to the environment to solve environmental problems, but these solutions carried additional problems of their own.

The insecticide DDT was once thought to be a completely benign substance; it is relatively nontoxic to humans and other mammals. At one time, DDT was used worldwide to eradicate malaria by killing the mosquitoes that carry this dangerous disease. A study by the National Academy of Sciences stated that "in a little more than two decades, DDT prevented 500 million deaths that otherwise would have been inevitable," and the World Health Organization claimed that DDT had "killed more insects and saved more humans than any other substance." It was eventually discovered, however, that exposure to DDT caused birds to develop very thin egg shells, such that baby chicks did not hatch, and the bird population, particularly that of eagles, rapidly decreased. DDT kills hatching birds by interfering with their hormone balance. This environmental problem is caused by two phenomena: by the potentiating effect of DDT which increases the concentration of an enzyme that inactivates the bird's hormones, and by mimicking female hormones called estrogens. The balance between saving the lives of wild birds versus those of children threatened by malaria becomes a difficult tradeoff when deciding whether to use DDT in a poor, tropical country.

Other environmental chemicals can also act as weak estrogens in humans. For example, industrial chemicals known as polychlorinated biphenyls, or PCBs, accumulate in body fat, in which they are soluble. Because of their weak estrogenic activity and the fact that the more estrogen a woman is exposed to, the greater her risk of breast cancer, it was suggested that exposure to these estrogen mimics might have contributed to the slow rise in the incidence of breast cancer in the United States. Such issues can be explored only by epidemiologic studies, because it is unethical to conduct these types of experiments on humans. A large, well-designed epidemiologic study of the relationship between the levels of DDT and PCBs and the incidence of breast cancer was completed in 1997. The results indicate that these two chemicals are extremely unlikely to be linked to breast cancer. This outcome is not too surprising, for it had long been known that plants contain many naturally occurring estrogens. The amount of biologically active plant estrogens in a single glass of red wine is 1,000 times greater than all of the environmental chemicals that an individual would ingest from pesticides in a day's food. Many more natural plant estrogens enter the body from vegetables in the diet than from environmental chemicals.

Bisphenol A, a synthetic chemical that is a polymer plasticizer, is claimed to act as an estrogen mimic in mice. This compound is so widely used that everyone in the industrialized world has been exposed to it. Bisphenol A can leach from dental sealants and food-can linings and from polycarbonate bottles and dishes. About 1.6 billion pounds of this substance are produced each year in the United States. No one knows whether humans ingest enough bisphenol A to cause adverse health effects, but this question is being studied.

Malathion is an insecticide that is occasionally in the news. This synthetic chemical is sometimes used to control insects. In unusual circumstances, malathion has been sprayed from aircraft, for example, in California to limit infestations of fruit flies, which threaten large agricultural regions, and in New York City to curb mosquitoes that may carry a deadly form of encephalitis. In humans and other mammals, malathion is mildly toxic. Its toxicity depends on the animal and the dose. Malathion is moderately toxic to birds and can be highly toxic to fish such as walleye pike and trout, but it is less toxic to goldfish. In most cases, malathion is detoxified by metabolism in the animal and is rapidly eliminated through urine, feces, and expired air. Malathion breaks down fairly rapidly in soil and ground water, such that it has a low persistence in the environment. Insects, and to a lesser extent fish, do not detoxify malathion as rapidly as mammals do; for this reason, malathion is much more toxic to insects than to mammals and is a potent insecticide. Malathion spraying poses a classic risk–benefit situation. Sometimes the public good outweighs the slight health hazard present and the public's fear of chemicals. These decisions are often more political than scientific.

Malathion is a neurotoxin that acts by inhibiting cholinesterase, an enzyme necessary for nerve function. Similar organophosphate human-enzyme inhibitors are much more slowly degraded, and these can be extremely toxic to humans. An example is the nerve gas sarin, which is 26 times more lethal than hydrogen cyanide gas—a pinprick-sized droplet would kill you. Sarin strongly inhibits cholinesterase, resulting in convulsions and paralysis of lung muscles.

Natural and Unnatural Molecules in the Environment

Sarin and related nerve gases are frightening terrorist weapons. Imagine sitting on a subway train and reading your newspaper. "Next stop, Grand Central," the conductor intones. Flipping the page, you think casually of the Yankee game, when suddenly your thought is interrupted by an uneasy feeling. Looking around, you see people foaming at the mouth and tears streaming from their eyes. Some are on the floor shaking. Your vision becomes dim, your nose starts to run, and your chest becomes tight. Soon, your breathing is irregular and shallow. Within minutes, you start to convulse. Death comes soon after. A similar nightmare happened in Japan on March 20, 1995, during morning rush hour. Although 5,500 commuters were affected, luckily, only 12 people died, because the sarin released by the Aum Supreme Truth cult was only 30% pure.

The Nazis discovered sarin, and, by the end of World War II, Germany had stockpiled more than 1,000 pounds of this nerve gas. It is a remarkable stroke of luck that, because Hitler had been gassed in World War I, the Germans never used any. Sarin is easy to make by combining two nontoxic chemicals. It is important to keep these chemicals away from terrorist groups and ruthless governments.

Gasoline additives

Gasoline additives are added to the environment for environmental reasons, but they can cause concern. An interesting case is methyl tertiary butyl ether (MTBE). This chemical has been added to gasoline to reduce the formation of carbon monoxide, which is emitted from the exhaust of older automobiles. MTBE was introduced into gasoline in 1992. By 1997, 31% of all gasoline in the United States contained MTBE; gasoline in California contained 11% MTBE! There is no better way to expose the public to a substance than to add it to gasoline. For example, in "breathing zones" around self-service gasoline pumps in some states (including California) that have vapor-recovery systems, median MTBE levels were 245 parts per billion (ppb), but in states without vapor controls, the median MTBE levels reached 1,500 ppb. Another problem is that, unlike most other fuel additives, MTBE is somewhat soluble in water and does not readily biodegrade. It has leaked into many wells, reservoirs, and lakes, thereby contaminating some of the water supply. The widespread contamination of water supplies in California is illustrated by the presence of 47 ppb of MTBE found in normally pristine Lake Tahoe and 9 ppb found in the Los Angeles water supply. The EPA has proposed a health-advisory level of 70 ppb, above which the public is advised to seek another source of drinking water. California's Department of Health places the recommended limit at 35 ppb. Most individuals can taste MTBE at concentrations above 40 ppb; many can taste it above 15 ppb. Is MTBE dangerous to human health at these levels? That is uncertain. Although rats and mice exposed to higher levels of MTBE developed various cancers, its human carcinogenic potency is not well understood. It is categorized as a "possible-to-probable human carcinogen."

Because this fuel additive had some environmental virtues in terms of automobile exhaust emission, various environmental advocacy groups lined up on both sides of this issue. A 1995 study showed that there is no difference in the total level of automobile toxic exhaust whether using reformulated fuel with or fuel without MTBE added. This is a good example of a multifaceted environmental problem involving economics, emotion, and politics all together. New cars, aided by automobile exhaust catalysts, can perform without serious emission problems, but political considerations rule out the removal of older cars by whatever means. By 1998, there was strong political pressure to remove MTBE from gasoline, and by 1999, its use was beginning to be phased out.

In the early 1920s, two agents were considered as "antiknock" additives to gasoline: tetraethyllead and ethanol. Although known to be toxic, tetraethyllead was chosen for financial reasons—it could be patented, whereas ethanol could not! Executives at DuPont, which controlled 36% of General Motors stock, and at GM chose to produce the more lucrative, but nevertheless toxic, tetraethyllead. From 1923 to 1986, 7 million tons of this toxic additive were added to gasoline in the United States. Since 1976, when tetraethyllead began to be phased out to protect catalytic converters, blood-lead levels in the US population have declined 78%.

Ethanol (ethyl alcohol) has been proposed to replace the additive MTBE. This nontoxic, oxygenated additive is being promoted by powerful political, ecological, and industrial groups. Ethanol is produced by fermentation of agricultural crops, principally corn. When one accounts for the energy required to plant, harvest, and transport corn, and adds the energy used in fermentation and concentration of alcohol, many scientists estimate that the burning of ethanol in gasoline results in a net energy loss. It is also true that ethanol has less intrinsic energy than the hydrocarbon components in gasoline. Additional costs are associated with the use of ethanol because the production of corn is subsidized and because fuel containing alcohol, called gaso-hol, is subject to reduced taxes. One argument favoring gasohol use is that the ethanol additive is renewable, meaning that it is biological, or natural. The subsidies, the additional energy cost, and the fact that new cars do not need oxygenated additives are issues rarely discussed in the media. Nor does anyone mention the waste of an important pro-tein foodstuff by converting it into a fuel. In the farm states, because of the weak farm economy, political support for gasohol is very strong. Farm-state members of Congress do not want the oxygen requirement repealed; they want to mandate that ethanol be used as the chemical additive of choice. Large industries profit from the fermentation and concentration of ethanol to make gasohol, and these industries make substantial campaign contributions to politicians in both parties. Ecology-minded groups also advocate the use of ethanol in gasoline because it is renewable and natural. Laws supporting oxygenated ad-ditives in gasoline often specify that these additives must be renew-able. This restriction means that petroleum companies could not man-ufacture ethanol as a gasoline additive made from ethylene, a less-ex-pensive chemical made from petroleum and natural gas. Gasohol is not unsafe, but it is expensive and wasteful. There are additional com-plications. In California, requiring the use of ethanol would put 200 additional tank trucks on the road each day. It would also raise gaso-line prices by several cents a gallon. Finally, you may not know that the major components in gasoline are themselves toxic, especially so called aromatic hydrocarbons. The latter are mild carcinogens. Thus, pumping your own gasoline is a risky activity.

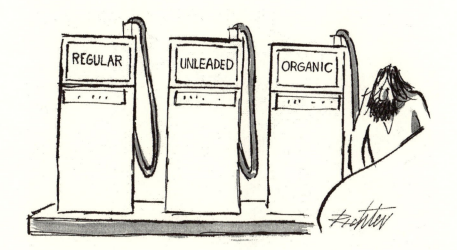

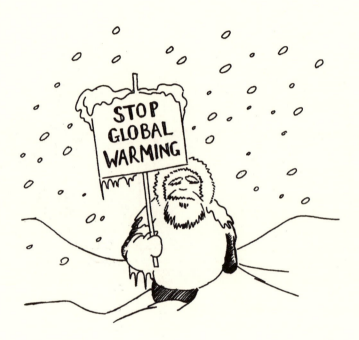

CHAPTER

8

Is the Sky Falling??

REMEMBER THE FABLE in which Chicken Little asked if "the sky is falling"? In the media, there is a lot of discussion about the atmosphere and whether human activities are causing environmental pollution of the sky. Is the sky falling? Consider, for example, a mystery discussed on late-night talk radio about the contrails left behind by high-flying airplanes. Some callers claimed that these made people sick! This contrail controversy reached epidemic proportions on the internet. Of course, this concept is nonsense; the term *contrail* is a contraction for "condensation trail" and refers simply to the water vapor in a plane's exhaust that condenses in the upper atmosphere. Contrails are formed above 30,000 feet, where the air temperature is between 20 and 40 degrees below zero, so that the water condenses into ice crystals. The same crystals can be seen on most sunny days as the cirrus clouds we can see in the sky. There is no danger from contrails or clouds, but as you will see below, some human-caused pollution in the atmosphere may pose real problems.

Acid Rain

Every other week, it seems, a news report appears concerning acid rain. What *is* acid rain, what causes it, and what harm does it do? The term *acid rain* refers to pollutants in clouds resulting from both natural sources and human activities. The formation of acid rain is illustrated in Figure 14. Certain gases including nitrogen dioxide (NO_2), sulfur dioxide (SO_2), and sulfur trioxide (SO_3) are dehydrated forms of acids. When exposed to water vapor, these gases react and

169

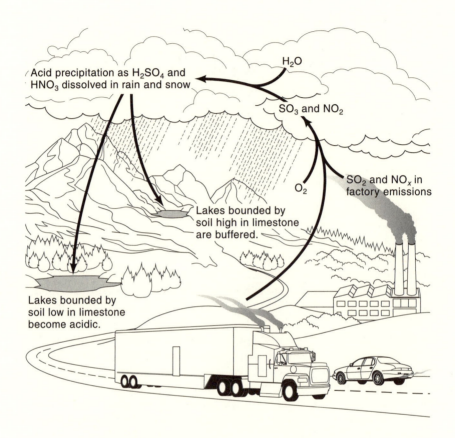

Figure 14. Mechanism of acid rain formation.

become strong acids: nitric (HNO$_3$) and sulfuric (H$_2$SO$_4$) acids. To achieve their maximum acidity, sulfur dioxide and nitrogen dioxide first need to react with oxygen in the air, but this occurs readily. The acidic sulfur oxides, SO$_2$ and SO$_3$, come from burning elemental sulfur in fuels such as soft coal and unrefined petroleum, as well as from natural volcanic emissions—even hot-springs emit SO$_2$. Nitrogen oxides are formed during the combustion of fuels in power plants and especially in automobiles. This reaction occurs because nitrogen gas (N$_2$), a major component of air, readily burns at the high temperatures of furnaces and automobile engines to form NO and NO$_2$ (these are collectively called NO$_x$). In air, these nitrogen oxide gases are even-

Is the Sky Falling??

Table 8   The pH values of various rainwaters compared with those of common acids

Source	pH
Normal rainwater (contains CO_2)	5.6
Average US rainwater	4.1
Pennsylvania and Sweden rainwater	2.7
Wheeling, West Virginia, rainwater	1.8
Acidic fog in California	1.6
Vinegar	2.7
Lemon juice	2.3
Stomach acid	2.0

tually transformed into nitric acid by reaction with water and oxygen. The same transformation occurs in lightning bolts, but the quantities of nitric acid formed in nature are small compared with those from human sources. Acidic air is localized because it is produced by large power plants and then carried in particular directions by prevailing winds. Acidity is measured on a logarithmic pH scale. Neutral solutions are neither acidic nor basic; their pH values are 7. Acidic media have pH values lower than 7; solutions with pH values higher than 7 are basic. Like the Richter scale used to measure the strength of earthquakes, each pH unit represents a 10-fold change in acidity or basicity. Table 8 lists the pH values recorded for various rainwaters and shows, for comparison, the pH values of common acids. Figure 15 shows a diagram of familiar aqueous solutions across all the pH values.

Far downwind from the source of pollution, acid rain from these sources destroys trees and kills fish. Acid rain kills trees by releasing aluminum salts from the soil, which increases the soil's acidity (Figure 16, see color section). This result is especially evident in Germany's Black Forest. Many sorts of fish are sensitive to pH changes; some species die in water with pH values between pH 4.5 and 5.0. Acid rain is thought to be responsible for declining fish

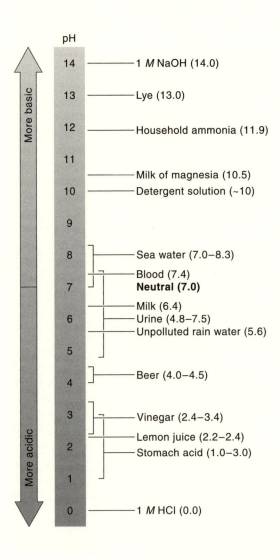

Figure 15. The pH values of some common aqueous solutions.

populations in several parts of the world. For example, trout populations are reduced in slightly acidic rivers. By comparison, trout prosper in slightly alkaline streams such as the Crooked River in western Oregon.

Because of environmental damage from acid rain, major efforts have been made to remove NO_x from auto exhausts and from the stack gases of power plants. There are also regulations to use low-sulfur fuels in gasoline and in power plants to reduce sulfur dioxide emissions. Complying with these environmental regulations is expensive and sometimes resisted by power companies and occasionally by the public. Such environmental regulations can sometimes have unfortunate consequences, illustrating the complexity of environmental science. For example, curbing sulfur emissions from power plants across northern Europe had the unanticipated result of killing agricultural crops! Apparently, while many plants do not like acid, they do require sulfur, and some farmland is sulfur-deficient. One method of solving that problem is to use ammonium sulfate, $(NH_4)_2(SO_4)$, as a fertilizer. This substance provides both nitrogen and sulfur, which are essential plant nutrients.

Other environmental fixes for combating acid rain are impractical. For example, one way to modify the effect of acid rain on a lake would be to add a base to neutralize the acids in the lake; lime is the cheapest strong base. Such treatment, however, is prohibitively expensive because of the huge volume of water that would have to be treated. For example, in Canada the cost of raising the pH has been estimated to be $50 per acre of lake; within a few years, a treated lake would again become acidic and require retreatment. There is no free lunch in the solution of this problem—every solution is costly.

Global Warming and the Greenhouse Effect

There appears to be a problem with the sky, and many people claim it is because of human activities. The media frequently feature stories about global warming resulting from a phenomenon called the greenhouse effect. In 1998, the mean surface temperature of the globe reached 0.58° C (approximately 1° F) above the average temperature for the period 1961 through 1990, making 1998 the warmest year since at least 1860. Continued projected increases in the Earth's temperature would cause immense problems, because the ice caps at the North and South Poles might melt to some extent, and low coastal regions, such as those around the San Francisco Bay and New Orleans, would be flooded. Weather patterns around the Earth might also change, resulting in more violent weather. What is this concern all about? Is the current global warming a long-term phenomenon, or just a fluctuation over a few decades? Is this change the result of human activities? What is the science behind global warming? Global warming is a very complex subject, one that not all scientists agree about. It has become a controversial, even political, topic. After you have read the following overview, you may be able to better interpret arguments in the media about global warming.

We can start by understanding that the greenhouse phenomenon results from the interaction of sunlight with particular gases in the Earth's atmosphere. This interaction causes these so-called greenhouse gases to act like an insulating blanket and retain some of the warmth that comes from sunlight. The "blanket" of greenhouse gases amplifies the effect of the solar heating that comes from visible and ultraviolet light. This effect is illustrated in Figure 17. All of the gases in the sky are transparent to solar radiation in the visible and ultraviolet regions and let this energetic light through, much like a window pane transmits sunlight to warm a room. The heat generated by sunlight on the Earth's surface is converted into infrared radiation, which is emitted back out into space. Part of this emitted infrared radiation is absorbed by greenhouse gases in the atmosphere, and part is reflected back to the Earth, warming the surface. The remainder of this infrared radiation escapes into outer space. Your eye cannot see infrared light, but infrared light from a fire or another heat source can be felt warming your body. This invisible infrared light is sometimes referred to as heat waves. In the atmosphere, greenhouse gases absorb some of this emitted infrared light. Not all of the gases in the atmosphere are greenhouse gases; for example, oxygen and nitrogen are not, and those molecules do not absorb infrared light. The greenhouse gases absorb in different regions of the infrared spectral window, depending on the particular greenhouse gas.

Virtually all scientists agree that the greenhouse phenomenon is real. Without these greenhouse gases, the Earth would have an average temperature of -18° C (-0.4° F) rather than the actual present average temperature of 15° C (59° F). In the absence of the Earth's atmosphere, human life would not be possible because of the low temperatures. The climates of two other planets illustrate the importance

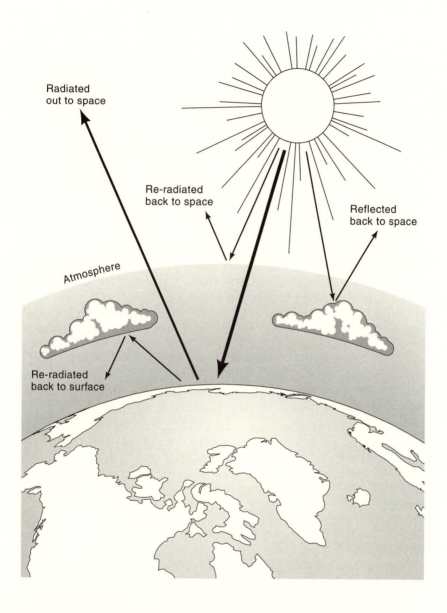

Figure 17. The role of the atmosphere in maintaining the surface temperature of the Earth. Solar radiation is partially reflected back into space, and partially absorbed by the atmosphere; some reaches the surface, mostly as visible light. Both the surface and the atmosphere re-radiate part of the absorbed energy as heat (infrared radiation), which is either lost in space or is captured by clouds and greenhouse gases.

of the greenhouse phenomenon. Mars has almost no atmosphere and is consequently very cold, because its heat is radiated to outer space. In contrast, Venus has a thick blanket of a greenhouse gas, carbon dioxide, which retains so much heat that Venus is very hot, more than 500° C, hot enough to melt lead. Because of these temperature extremes, neither planet can support life as we know it. Taking all this information into consideration, is there a greenhouse problem on Earth, and is it caused by human activities? It is true that some greenhouse gases are increasing as the result of human activities; thus, we *may* face the prospect of an increasing temperature on Earth.

It is certain that the sky can affect the temperature. For example, you know that a clear winter night becomes a lot colder than a cloudy one; the water vapor in the clouds has a greenhouse effect by capturing and re-radiating infrared energy back to the earth. Cloudless deserts become very cold at night because the dry air absorbs no infrared radiation, and heat is lost as infrared radiation to outer space.

The effect of clouds complicates mathematical modeling of the greenhouse phenomenon. During the day, clouds may shield the Earth from the warming sunlight, so less energy from sunlight gets through. Clouds that are contaminated with sulfuric acid droplets (from a volcano or power plants burning sulfur-rich brown coal) are especially effective in blocking sunlight. A dramatic example of this phenomenon is illustrated by aftereffects from the huge eruption of the Indonesian volcano, Tambora, in 1815; the ash and sulfuric acid droplets caused temperatures to drop around the world. For example, in the region around Ohio, temperatures that year fell below freezing in mid-July. The violence of the Tambora volcano was huge, 50 times that of the St. Helens eruption in Washington State in May, 1980.

The greenhouse gases

What are the different greenhouse gases? Some, such as carbon dioxide, may be familiar to you, but you may be surprised by others that are usually not identified in the media. What property distinguishes a greenhouse gas? A greenhouse gas molecule absorbs infrared energy because stretching of its bonds causes a separation of positive and negative charges. Scientists would describe this stretching by saying the dipole moment of these bonds changes when they vibrate. These bond stretches are like notes in a piano; they occur at different tones or frequencies. Non-greenhouse molecules such as oxygen and

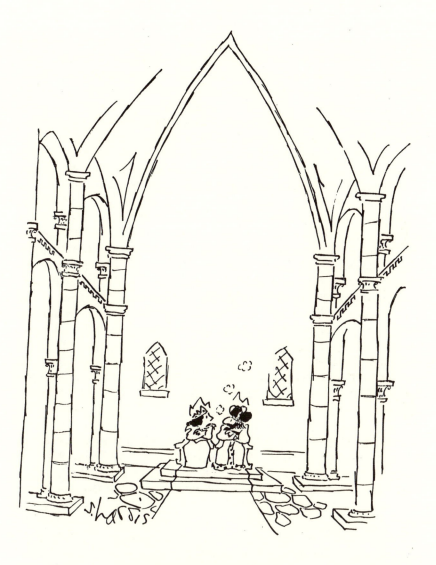

"IF I'VE LEARNED ONE THING IN MY LONG REIGN, IT'S THAT HEAT RISES."

Is the Sky Falling??

nitrogen, which make up most of the atmosphere, do not have this property of charge separation and do not absorb infrared light. The important greenhouse gases—water vapor, carbon dioxide, methane, Freons, and laughing gas—are described below.

Water vapor. Most of the public does not realize that the major greenhouse gas is water vapor! The amount of water vapor in the air varies according to atmospheric conditions. This lack of consistency complicates calculations of the greenhouse phenomenon. Some calculations indicate that more than 97% of the greenhouse effect is caused by water vapor. The amount of water vapor in the air depends on the temperature and the altitude at that part of the Earth. Wherever the air is very cold, the concentration of water vapor is low. If the air is very cold, the ground may also be coated with snow or ice. Conversely, if the air is warm, as it is in the atmosphere over tropical oceans, the concentration of water vapor will be higher because of increased evaporation. As water evaporates from lakes or the sea, the Earth cools. Remember that water drops in clouds also cool the Earth by shielding the sun and reflecting solar radiation. On the other hand, water vapor is a significant greenhouse gas that warms the Earth. Clearly, calculations of the heat balance involving water can get very complicated. The effect of clouds is sometimes ignored, especially by those who argue that there is a serious greenhouse problem.

Carbon dioxide. Carbon dioxide is the greenhouse gas that is much in the news; after water vapor, it accounts for much of the remaining greenhouse warming. The concentration of carbon dioxide in the atmosphere has been steadily increasing since the Industrial Revolution as a result of human activities such as the combustion of fossil fuels; the graph in Figure 18 clearly illustrates this phenomenon. This evidence is the "smoking gun" used in arguments favoring anthropological effects on global warming.

Because the global analysis of carbon dioxide in the atmosphere has been made only recently, how, you might ask, do we know that carbon dioxide levels in the air have been increasing over many years? In fact, the historical analysis of atmospheric carbon dioxide graphed in Figure 18 was carried out by drilling deep ice cores in polar regions such as Greenland. These ice cores represent a time record; the concentration of carbon dioxide and ratios of oxygen isotopes in the ice are measured along the entire core. In Greenland,

Is the Sky Falling??

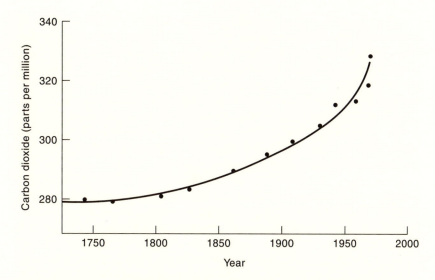

Figure 18. Carbon dioxide concentrations in the air within glacier bubbles have steadily increased over the past 250 years.

each year's snowfall is compacted into ice, trapping air bubbles. This water carries an isotopic "fingerprint" of temperature records in past times. The isotopic content of ice is determined by the temperature of the snow as it forms and falls. From these tree-ring-like ice cores, scientists have a record of the gases present in the atmosphere over Greenland and of the changes in the air temperature over the past 250,000 years—a period that covers the last two major ice ages.

How has the concentration of CO_2 over the Earth's atmosphere changed over very long time periods? During the time of the dinosaurs, 100 million years ago, the carbon dioxide concentration was more than 1,000 parts per million, whereas the value before the Industrial Revolution hovered near 280 ppm, less than one-third as much. In 1998, the CO_2 level had increased to about 360 ppm.

Let's consider some natural sources of CO_2. An interesting example of natural production is the carbon dioxide emitted at Yellowstone National Park, an area rich in mudpots, geysers, and other volcanic activity. The entire park is estimated to give off 44 million tons of carbon dioxide each year, roughly 10 times the annual amount released by a medium sized power plant burning fossil fuels.

Is the Sky Falling??

Another CO_2 source in nature comes from all animals, including ourselves, who consume plant products and animal proteins. After extracting the energy from these plant and animal products through respiration (reaction of the products with oxygen), we exhale carbon dioxide as a byproduct (Figure 19, see color section). This process is a minor contribution to the total amount of carbon dioxide in the atmosphere. Of course, plant forms of all types (from rain forests, algae, grass, etc.) constantly consume carbon dioxide from the air, converting it into carbohydrates and releasing oxygen—a non-greenhouse gas that we need for life.

The major anthropologic source of carbon dioxide is the combustion of fossil fuels (petroleum, natural gas, and coal). The burning of fossil fuels is a measure of society's energy production and consumption. These fossil fuels are photosynthetic products that have accumulated over millions of years; the sun's energy produced them in green plants by transforming carbon dioxide from the air into carbohydrates. Burning these fossil fuels regenerates energy and turns the former plant products back into carbon dioxide. The rise in atmospheric carbon dioxide comes from our increasing use of the finite amounts of fossil fuels presently on Earth. The amount of carbon dioxide generated by the average person throughout the world is about 1 ton per year; in developed western countries, this figure is much higher. For instance, each person in the United States generates five times the world average. As countries become more prosperous, the amount of energy required per capita increases, putting a greater burden on the limited supplies of fossil fuels and releasing more carbon dioxide into the atmosphere, which is thought to add to greenhouse warming. Additional fossil fuel energy is also needed to produce the food required to feed the increasing world population. The only major alternative to energy production without generating carbon dioxide is atomic energy. The people who are the most concerned about curtailing carbon dioxide production are, generally speaking, also opposed to the use of atomic energy. This is a good example of tough choices illustrating the principle, "there is no free lunch."

Figure 20 (see color section) shows the global carbon cycle. The amounts of carbon dioxide being taken up and given off are presented in green and red, respectively. These figures are listed in gigatons of carbon per year. These amounts are huge; *giga* stands for 10^9, a thousand million. Only 5 out of a total of 197 gigatons of carbon given off from all sources (plants, soil, ocean, etc.) are derived from the burning of fossil fuels (coal, oil, natural gas, and gasoline). This share of carbon dioxide from human activities is only about 3% of the total! This 3% is the quantity that the Global Warming Treaty proposes to reduce or minimize.

The time a greenhouse gas remains in the atmosphere is important in measuring its greenhouse effect over long periods of time. This time depends on the rate required for a quantity of carbon dioxide to return to the Earth's surface. Scientists call this rate a half-life. The rate at which the oceans remove carbon dioxide from the atmosphere depends in part on the temperature. In the same way that a carbonated drink gives off its carbon dioxide when warm and remains fizzy when cold, warmer oceans take up less carbon dioxide than cold oceans do. On average, a substantial fraction of a carbon dioxide sample stays in the atmosphere for a century. This means that some carbon dioxide from the coal that kept President McKinley warm is still "up there." Other greenhouse gases do not stay in the atmosphere for such a long period. These gases have faster rates of return, or conversion. For example, methane reacts with oxygen in the air and is converted into carbon dioxide.

There is another problem with the carbon dioxide greenhouse phenomenon that is seldom discussed in the media; even most scientists are unaware of it. Within the frequency range in which carbon dioxide absorbs infrared radiation, most of the radiation being given off from the Earth is already being absorbed by the carbon dioxide now present in the atmosphere. In other words, the greenhouse effect of carbon dioxide is nearly "maxed out." Some higher vibrational states (so-called hot bands) and some fringes of the carbon dioxide spectrum remain to absorb additional infrared radiation. This means that if the carbon dioxide in the atmosphere were to increase—even by a lot—the corresponding amount of heat absorbed by it would not increase by as much because the change is not proportionate. Other types of greenhouse gases such as methane, Freons, nitrous oxide, and water, however, are not "maxed-out." Of these, methane is the most potent and unpredictable because of the unstable stores of methane, termed methane ice, trapped in the deep oceans.

Methane. The major constituent of natural gas, methane, is another important greenhouse gas whose concentration is increasing because of human activities. By sampling Arctic ice of known ages, scientists learned that the methane concentration in the atmosphere remained constant for nearly 30,000 years and then began to increase toward the end of the 17th century; at present, it is increasing more rapidly and has doubled over the past 200 years. Actually, even though the amount of methane in the Earth's atmosphere is not very high (about 1/200th that of carbon dioxide), methane is 20 to 25 times more potent than CO_2 as an absorber of infrared energy. Some estimates indicate that, ignoring water vapor, methane accounts for about 18% of the increase in the total greenhouse effect. Because methane persists in the atmosphere for only about 10 years, cuts in methane emissions would rapidly reduce global concentrations. In contrast, you may remember that atmospheric carbon dioxide lasts from 5 to 20 times as long—about a century.

We have considerable potential for adding large amounts of methane to the atmosphere. Leaking gas wells, coal mines, and decaying garbage dumps all contribute to the methane in the atmosphere. Russian gas pipelines and wellheads leak an estimated 35 million tons of methane into the atmosphere each year. Termites also produce large quantities of methane; an estimated 20% of atmospheric methane comes from termites. Methane is also produced in large quantities by bacteria in the innards of cows and sheep. In Great Britain, approximately 23% of the released methane can be traced to belching and farting cattle. Sheep, pigs, poultry, horses, and people account for another 10%. As mentioned earlier, each person gives forth between 300 and 2,000 ml per day in this way. An acceleration of greenhouse warming could occur from the sum of these sources.

The largest potential source of methane gas might arise from solid hydrates of methane that are stable only at low temperatures and high pressures. Scientists believe that this methane ice may contain twice as much energy as all the world's sources of oil, coal, and natural gas combined. Methane ice is located in immense deposits under deep oceans, where it is stabilized by low temperatures and high pressures, and also under the permafrost in the Arctic. Methane hydrate packs methane so efficiently that 164 cubic feet of methane gas can be squeezed into a single cubic foot of methane hydrate. At present, there is no economic method to mine or harvest this energy source.

Freons. Among the worst synthetic greenhouse gases are the so-called Freons, which are chlorofluorocarbons used as refrigerants in refrigerators and air-conditioners. On a per-molecule basis, these very stable gases can be 10,000 times as effective as carbon dioxide in absorbing infrared radiation. There are two reasons for their effectiveness. Their carbon–fluorine bonds have very intense infrared stretching bands; these bonds absorb nearly all the infrared radiation at wavelengths corresponding to their vibrations. These wavelengths reside in a region of the spectrum in which none of the other greenhouse gases exhibits infrared absorption. Later in this chapter, you will learn that these chlorofluorocarbons are also catalytic killers of atmospheric ozone and thereby create the ozone hole. Unfortunately, the residence time of Freons in the atmosphere is about 10 times longer than that of methane, so the Freons are also more persistent greenhouse gases than methane.

Nitrous oxide, laughing gas. Another of the greenhouse gases that contributes to global warming is nitrous oxide, the so-called laughing gas used as an anesthetic by dentists. This molecule is about 200 times more effective than carbon dioxide at trapping heat (infrared) radiation in the atmosphere. The largest known sources of nitrous oxide are emissions from bacteria in the soil and the ocean, fertilizer decomposition, combustion, and industrial processes such as nylon manufacture. Nitrous oxide is so unreactive that it easily escapes from the surface of the Earth and diffuses into the upper atmosphere.

Other natural causes of global warming

Global warming may not be caused entirely by the greenhouse gases. Another possible culprit is the sun. The periodic rhythms of sunspots and flares appearing in cycles of about 11 years could account for much of the global warming to date. Sunspots are dark patches that occur on the sun's surface. Sunspots are actually cooler areas that appear dark only because we observe them against a brighter background. The number of spots increases and decreases with time in a regular cycle that covers about 11 years. Some aspects of weather seem to be synchronized with sunspot activity. Events in the sun that cause sunspots are correlated with a slightly higher energy output.

This phenomenon is illustrated in Figure 21. The viewpoint that much of global warming is associated with sunspot cycles is strongly contested by many environmental activists, who insist that the greenhouse gases are mostly to blame. Surprisingly, the sun is at its brightest when sunspots are at a peak. During these periods, the sun provides the greatest warmth to the Earth. Other factors affecting global warming are also involved in conjunction with the sunspots. For ex-

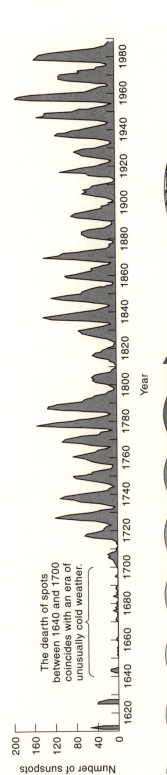

The dearth of spots between 1640 and 1700 coincides with an era of unusually cold weather.

Number of sunspots

200
160
120
80
40
0

1620 1640 1660 1680 1700 1720 1740 1760 1780 1800 1820 1840 1860 1880 1900 1920 1940 1960 1980

Year

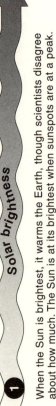 **Solar brightness**

When the Sun is brightest, it warms the Earth, though scientists disagree about how much. The Sun is at its brightest when sunspots are at a peak.

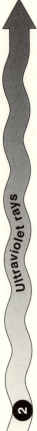 **Ultraviolet rays**

Brightness means more ultraviolet radiation, which produces more ozone in the upper atmosphere. These changes are linked to shifts in storm patterns.

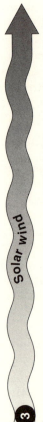 **Solar wind**

Solar winds of ionized hydrogen and helium particles block cosmic rays, making the atmosphere less conductive and thus discouraging cloud formation and precipitation.

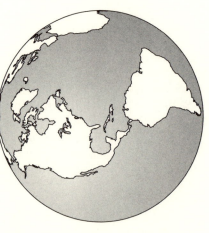

Figure 21. The Earth's temperature correlates with the abundance of sunspots.

184

ample, the brightness yields more ultraviolet rays, which produce more ozone in the upper atmosphere. The magnetic solar wind, composed of ionized hydrogen and helium atoms, is also at a maximum during these periods. Solar winds block cosmic rays, which would otherwise stimulate rainfall. Obviously, this phenomenon is all very complex and difficult to model, even with supercomputers, thereby leaving a lot of room for controversy.

You may ask: what is the evidence connecting past episodes of sunspots with temperature variation? Of course, sunspots can be observed through telescopes, but there are other methods of historical analysis. For example, the time record of cosmic rays can be followed by analyzing the isotope carbon-14 in tree rings. Cosmic rays produce this strange carbon-14 isotope that rains down and is eventually incorporated into tree rings, thus giving a detailed history of solar activity. A dramatic correlation is found between diminished sunspot activity and cooling of the Earth. In the "Little Ice Age" shown in Figure 21 between 1640 and 1720, the number of sunspots fell sharply, and the Earth cooled about two degrees Fahrenheit, compared with the estimated warming of roughly one degree between 1880 and the present. This 17th century period strongly affected northern Europe, as its glaciers grew and winters lengthened.

The Greenland ice core data give evidence for abrupt changes in the global climate. Some scientists speculate that our current global warming could actually trigger an abrupt *cooling* that might occur too quickly to make adjustments in agriculture. Europe's climate might become more like Siberia's. The last time an abrupt cooling occurred was in the midst of a period of global warming. The mechanism for such sudden temperature changes involves the circular ocean currents, which redistribute heat; for example, equatorial heat is carried to the temperate zones. The relative salt concentrations in seawater affect these currents because saltier water is heavier and sinks. The oceans are not well mixed, but the phenomenon of mixing produces giant oceanic currents that influence the global climate. For example, salt water sinking in the Nordic Seas causes warm water to flow farther north than it might otherwise do. This phenomenon accounts for the winters in northern Europe being milder than would be predicted from the latitude. These factors are very complex and are also difficult to model with computers.

From analysis of ancient ocean sediments, there is evidence of wild climatic variations over the past 10,000 years. Episodes of warmth, cold, drought, and flooding have been much more extreme than anything experienced in the 20th century. For example, about 1,000 years ago, Europe basked in warmth that nurtured vineyards in Britain and allowed the Vikings to colonize Greenland. At the same time, California was experiencing century-long droughts. Only a few centuries later, severe cold gripped the Earth in the Little Ice Age. Europe froze, crops failed, and glaciers advanced. There is strong evidence for pervasive, natural climatic changes that occur more or less regularly about every 1,500 years, resulting in centuries-long cold spells much like the Little Ice Age. These periodic swings have occurred over 32,000 years, which is as far back as the ocean sediments can be dated by the radiocarbon dating method. These natural, periodic temperature swings, which are not understood, raise important questions in the current scientific debate over global warming and the greenhouse phenomenon. How much of the temperature change that has occurred over the past century has been caused by waste industrial gases that trap heat in the atmosphere?

One suggestion of a possible mechanism by which the Earth might have recovered from past ice ages is the melting of naturally occurring methane hydrates and the release of the powerful greenhouse gas methane. During the last ice age, which ended about 12,000 years ago, sea levels dropped about 300 feet (the length of a football field). It has been proposed that the lower sea levels reduced the pressure on the gas hydrates so that these solids melted, releasing huge quantities of methane. Through the greenhouse phenomenon, the released methane may have helped warm the atmosphere and shift climatic gears to a warmer climate.

The exact progress of greenhouse warming is difficult to calculate. The rate at which the oceans remove carbon dioxide from the atmosphere depends in part on the temperature. The contributions of clouds and the uptake of carbon dioxide by tiny plants in the ocean are only two of many factors. The temperatures in the troposphere (lower atmosphere) may have been decreasing slightly as the temperature on the surface of the Earth has been increasing. No one seems to understand this temperature difference, but in 1998, a reanalysis of the satellite data indicated that this difference may not be very great. Measurements from more than 5,000 weather stations around the Earth indicate that between 1950 and 1993, night-time warming has been greater than daytime warming. Increased cloudiness could explain this trend because clouds reduce daytime but raise night-time temperatures. By 1997, most scientists agreed that there had been some increase in the global temperature from the greenhouse phenomenon, but the long-range, extrapolated temperature rise is not at all known at the moment; neither are there any inexpensive "quick fixes" to this long-range phenomenon.

You can understand that the greenhouse phenomenon is complicated and difficult to model mathematically, even with supercomputers. The reason is not that the supercomputers are not fast enough but that many equations must be formulated to account for all of the sometimes-conflicting features in this complex issue. For example, a major difficulty with these mathematical models concerns how to treat water vapor in the atmosphere, which increases with increasing temperature. Recall that some people believe this effect will enhance greenhouse warming because water is a greenhouse gas, but others note that cloud formation resulting from water vapor would have the opposite effect, except at night.

Calculations of the greenhouse phenomenon are further complicated by natural feedback mechanisms, which can be positive or negative. An example of negative feedback, in which a process limits itself automatically, occurs when a column of warm air rising from a warm region on the Earth's surface encounters cold air. The resulting condensation would produce a cloud, and the cloud would reduce the amount of sunlight heating the surface, thereby cooling the initially warm region. An example of positive feedback occurs when sunlight shines through a crack in an ice floe onto ocean water. Unlike ice, which reflects sunlight back into space, the ocean water absorbs most of the solar radiation that reaches it and warms up, exposing more water to the sun. Thus, cold, reflective ice fields can become warmed if the ice begins to fracture. The increased water vapor adds more greenhouse gas, which could further raise the temperature.

Computer models calculating the greenhouse effect are still no more than cloudy crystal balls (forgive the pun). Although cloud influences pose problems, the most modern computer programs do attempt to include the effect of tiny solid and liquid particles in the atmosphere called aerosols. Aerosols are composed primarily of sulfur dioxide droplets emitted by industry or by volcanoes. For example, in 1991, the Philippine volcano Mount Pinatubo erupted, sending aloft a global haze of aerosols. A calculation successfully predicted cooling of about one degree for a period of two years. Scientists are now attempting to include in their models deep-ocean processes that are also critical to analysis of the Earth's climate. This aspect is complex because the ocean absorbs both carbon dioxide and heat, transports heat to other regions, and provides moisture (the major greenhouse gas) to the atmosphere.

Concern over global warming lead to an international conference in Kyoto, Japan, in 1997. An agreement was reached that would mandate a 5% average global reduction in greenhouse gases. This deal included 38 of the world's most developed countries, including the United States, Japan, and the European Union. Different groups agreed to cut their greenhouse gas emissions by specified amounts over a 15-year period: the United States by 7%; Japan by 6%, and Europe by 8%. The United States Congress has yet to ratify this Kyoto Protocol, and no general agreement exists as to how the countries will accomplish these goals.

Various countries have developed local solutions to this worldwide issue. For example, a major anthropologic source of carbon dioxide comes from cement kilns, which now produce about 7% of the annual global CO_2 emissions. Producing 1 ton of cement releases 1 ton of CO_2. This activity is expected to reach 10% of the annual CO_2 production in the near future. Cement production creates CO_2 in two ways: by roasting limestone (calcium carbonate) inside the kilns, and by burning fossil fuels to heat the kilns to the very high temperatures necessary to drive off carbon dioxide to make calcium oxide. Yet the European Union proposals for a tax on energy aimed at reducing CO_2 production have excluded the cement industry for political reasons! Because of the Kyoto Protocol, Japan does not allow cement production in its country. But where do the Japanese get their cement? From Taiwan. Where does Taiwan get fuel to produce cement? From burning old rubber tires. Where does Taiwan get these tires? From the United States, where burning tires is discouraged because of pollution and carbon dioxide production. You can see that artificial economic and environmental distortions are being carried out in attempts to solve scientific problems politically.

Now you can see how global warming has become political. Some people fervently believe that global warming is an international crisis; others do not think this problem arises from human activities. On the one side, "the greens" are predicting disaster, but on the other, conservative radio talk-show host Rush Limbaugh says there is nothing to the problem. Environmental advocates and certain sympathetic politicians have made greenhouse warming a political issue. Their opponents say that, although there may be a greenhouse effect, it will only serve to ward off the next ice age! Both extremes stand on uncertain scientific foundations. In my opinion, this com-

THE FAR SIDE

By GARY LARSON

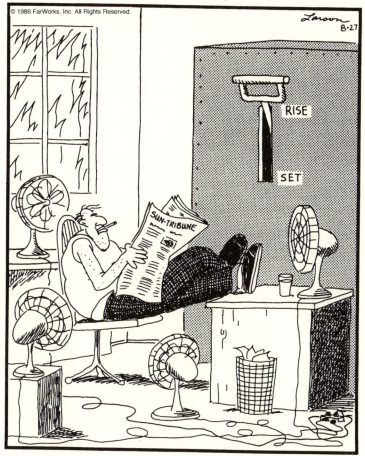

Inside the sun

plicated problem is still not fully resolved but does deserve additional study.

If there is a human-caused greenhouse problem, what could be done about it without disrupting the economy? The use of more energy-efficient devices such as fluorescent light bulbs is a good idea, but Americans' love for large cars is a bad idea. The only important energy sources that do not release CO_2 are hydroelectric and nuclear power, but both create other environmental problems. As usual with complex issues, the answers involve compromise.

The Ozone Hole

Many people are confused about ozone, a reactive form of oxygen. We are told that ozone is very toxic and must be kept at a low levels, especially in cities such as Los Angeles. But we are also told that there is an ozone "hole" in the upper atmosphere that is hazardous to life on the Earth. What is going on? Why do we need ozone one place but not another, and why is there too much ozone in one place and too little in another?

The upper atmosphere contains a thin layer of ozone, which has an important role in shielding animals and plants on Earth from the high-energy ultraviolet radiation coming from the sun. This small amount of ozone in the stratosphere acts to keep most of the sun's ultraviolet radiation from reaching the Earth. It is believed that life forms on Earth did not leave the protection of the sea to become established on land until the atmospheric ozone layer was established. Ozone (O_3) is an unstable form of ordinary oxygen (O_2). In the upper atmosphere, ultraviolet light provides the energy to transform oxygen into its less stable allotrope, ozone. Theoretically, ozone should revert to oxygen because the latter is more stable. Fortunately, this reaction is very slow; otherwise, the protective ozone layer in the upper atmosphere would vanish. Since about 1980, a dramatic decrease in the ozone concentration was found to occur over the South Pole during the early spring. This ozone hole has become a matter of worldwide concern. After extensive research and controversy, scientists have concluded that the major cause of the ozone depletion is a reaction for which chlorine atoms supported on the surface of tiny ice crystals act as the catalysts. The requirement that, to be an effective catalyst, the chlorine atoms must be supported on ice crystals explains the fact that ozone depletion is much more severe over the Antarctic than it is over the Arctic, because there are more ice crystals in the upper atmosphere over the Antarctic. The differences have to do with weather conditions such as a vortex of very cold air that forms over the South Pole in the southern winter. The stratosphere over Antarctica in winter is isolated by a circle of strong winds called the polar vortex such that in the winter, the ozone concentration remains stable. When the sun rises in early spring, dramatic ozone depletion occurs. In contrast, the arctic polar vortex is much weaker, and ozone concentrations in the north polar regions are constantly changing. In the mid-1990s, careful spectroscopic studies pointed to widespread catalytic destruction of Arctic ozone, which has been referred to as an ozone "dent." Beyond the polar regions, ozone depletion is also thought to be taking place, perhaps in small sulfate aerosol particles.

How do the chlorine atoms get into the upper atmosphere? Is this a new, anthropologic phenomenon? These catalytically active, ozone-destroying chlorine atoms principally result from the breakdown of certain normally very stable molecules called chlorofluorocarbons (CFCs). This breakdown takes place by action of the same high-energy ultraviolet radiation from which ozone protects the surface of the earth. The CFCs (also called Freons) are incredibly useful substances and are nontoxic to humans. These gases are widely employed in the compressors of most air-conditioners and refrigerators. They have also been used for cleaning computer chips and as propellants in spray cans. At its peak, worldwide production of CFCs reached about half a million tons per year. Unfortunately, because of their stability toward everything but ultraviolet light, the Freons have become widely distributed in the global atmosphere. It is estimated that each person on Earth now inhales several trillion CFC molecules with each breath! Even so, how can the CFC decomposition products have a substantial effect on the huge amount of ozone found in the upper atmosphere? The answer lies in the amplification or multiplication factor intrinsic to every catalytic process. Each chlorine atom is thought to catalyze the destruction of at least 100,000 ozone molecules!

The critical experiments that provided evidence that the CFCs threaten the Earth's protective ozone layer were performed by F. Sherwood Rowland (of the University of California, Irvine) and Mario Molina (of the Massachusetts Institute of Technology), starting

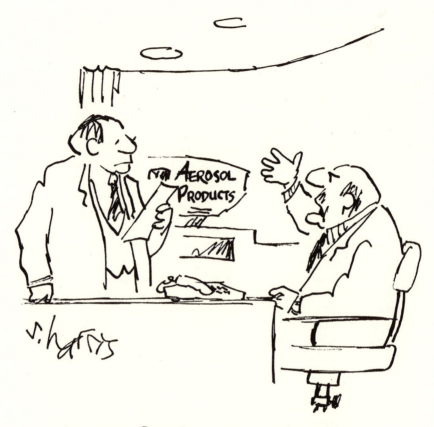

"OH, FOR PETE'S SAKE, LET'S JUST GET SOME OZONE AND SEND IT BACK UP THERE!"

in the 1970s. For many years, their controversial proposal was discounted, but strong experimental evidence eventually verified their hypothesis. Finally, in 1995, Rowland, Molina, and a German scientist, Paul Crutzen, were awarded the Nobel Prize for their research on ozone depletion. In 1987 an international agreement, the Montreal Protocol, was signed by many countries in an effort to control substances that deplete the ozone layer and to phase out the immensely useful CFCs. After extensive research, some chemical companies developed replacement refrigerant gases that do not generate chlorine atoms; however, these substitutes are not as effective as refrigerants and are more expensive than CFCs. If you have recently had your automobile air-conditioner recharged, you may be aware of this much greater cost. Freons, some of which can no longer be manufactured legally in the United States, have become a commodity illegally smuggled into the United States and other countries covered by the Montreal Protocol.

The average residence time of the CFCs in the atmosphere is about 100 years, as compared with the residence time of about 10 years for the greenhouse gas methane, which is easily oxidized. Because of the extraordinary stability of the CFCs and the catalytic amplification of ozone depletion by the chlorine atoms, it will be many years—well into this century—before ozone depletion is brought under control. In the interim, increased exposure to ultraviolet light will adversely affect both plant and animal life on at least some parts of the Earth. A 1% decrease in the tropospheric ozone is estimated to cause a 2% to 5% increase in incidence of treatable basal skin cancers and a 4% to 10% increase in incidence of the more dangerous squamous skin cancer.

In addition to the CFCs, other chemicals are also active in the catalytic destruction of ozone. One such "ozone eater" is bromine, which comes from agricultural chemicals, especially methyl bromide, a product used to spray strawberry fields. This molecule has a residence time of only about 10 months in the atmosphere. Another ozone destroyer is nitrous oxide (N_2O, laughing gas), used as an anesthetic gas in surgical and dental procedures. Most of the nitrous oxide in the atmosphere comes from naturally occurring biological processes, as in the decomposition of rotting vegetation. However, the concentration of this ozone-destroying gas has been increasing as a result of its large-scale production as a byproduct of nylon manufacturing. The major producers of nylon have voluntarily adopted procedures to prevent the escape of nitrous oxide into the atmosphere. Nitric oxide (NO), produced by subsonic and even more so by supersonic jet exhaust, also catalyzes ozone depletion. In the 1990s, there were fewer than 20 supersonic commercial aircraft (the European Concorde) in use, so this source is not yet a major problem. Solid propellants used by the space shuttle also introduce small amounts of chlorine into the atmosphere.

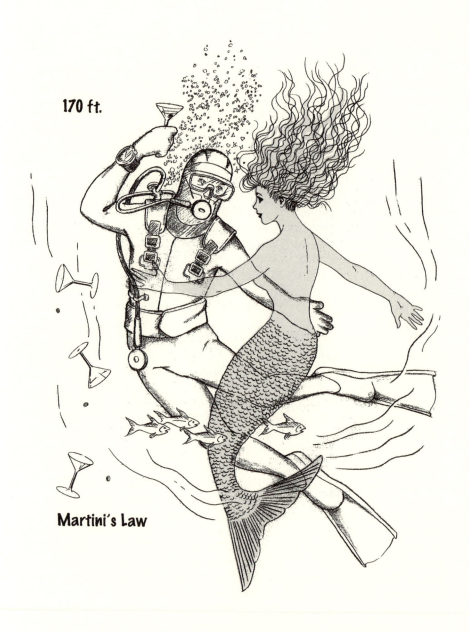

170 ft.

Martini's Law

Nitrogen Narcosis

9

Dust, Magnets, and Scuba Diving

Small Particles (Dust Can Be Dangerous)

A S SCIENTISTS HAVE LONG KNOWN, the presence of small particles in the air can be a health hazard, inducing emphysema and lung cancer. Some particles are dangerous because of their size, shape, and insolubility. Other small particles are also toxic because of their chemical nature; a familiar example is coal dust, which causes "black lung disease" in miners who breathe it in.

The most infamous particles are those from asbestos. Asbestos is a generic name for a variety of fibrous silicate minerals used for many purposes: in insulation for furnaces, buildings, and steam pipes; in textiles, concrete, and wall boards; for automobile brake pads and protective clothing worn by firefighters. The French emperor Charlemagne is supposed to have used a white tablecloth made from asbestos fibers; after a meal, the cloth was cleaned by burning off the food residues over a roaring fire! Asbestos has become a major cause of occupational lung disease. Asbestos abatement has become controversial. Removing asbestos from a structure is not only very expensive, but it may create a more hazardous situation because in the process of removing the asbestos, small particles may become airborne. Simply sealing over the insulation material may be cheaper and safer than removing it.

Dust, Magnets, and Scuba Diving

The most dangerous asbestos particles are needle-shaped, less than 0.1 micrometer in diameter, but more than 300 micrometers long (a ratio of 3,000 to 1). For comparison, a human hair is about 70 micrometers thick. Such long, thin asbestos particles can penetrate the alveoli, the sites in your lung where oxygen enters the bloodstream and carbon dioxide exits. Long-term exposure to asbestos is estimated to increase the risk of lung cancer by a factor of 5; for smokers, the risk is increased by another factor of 10. Many years ago, the Japanese polished their rice using asbestos; this practice is thought to have contributed to a high incidence of stomach cancer. This polishing procedure has long since been discontinued, and the incidence of stomach cancer has decreased.

There are two major types of asbestos: the insoluble carcinogenic fibers, called crodidolite, and the slightly soluble, apparently noncarcinogenic, curly crystals, called chrysotile. In the United States, about 95% of the asbestos used is chrysotile (white asbestos), but public fears of the term asbestos have resulted in a ban on all forms of asbestos and led to requirements that asbestos be removed from public buildings at a calculated cost ranging from $50 to $150 billion! Estimates are that on average, each person breathes in about one million asbestos fibers from natural geologic processes over a period of one year. The EPA has suggested that even a single asbestos fiber can cause cancer. A 1990 study of comparative risks, published in the journal *Science,* estimated that in a classroom used over a 5-year period, schoolchildren are 10 times more likely to die of complications from a whooping cough vaccination than they are to develop cancer from exposure to asbestos in that room. Whooping cough vaccination is often required for entry to school, a risk most people accept.

Even chemically benign particles can be dangerous if they are too small. People working in rock quarries or in grain elevators try to protect themselves from inhaling small particles, as do the Bedouins traveling in the desert. Throughout the 1800s and early 1900s, many workers exposed to silica died at an early age from silicosis, a fibrosis of the lungs. One study in the 1800s found that none of the workers in a factory in Sheffield, England, who used the silica grinding wheels survived beyond the age of 50!

My graduate students making chromatography columns wear masks to keep the fine silica particles from their lungs. However, similar silica particles are used to thicken ice cream! This use does not pose a problem, however, because we do not inhale ice cream;

there is a difference between putting something in your mouth and something in your nose, from where it can reach your lungs. I avoid jogging on a dry, crushed-rock road because of the small dust particles stirred up by passing cars. Even cotton lint from a clothes dryer is probably hazardous, and people should avoid breathing it.

Diesel-powered vehicles are more economical to use than gasoline-powered ones because they use less fuel. However, diesels pollute more. The black diesel fumes amount to about 150,000 tons annually in Europe. This diesel soot is less than 2.5 micrometers in diameter and is thought to penetrate deeply into the breathing passages, where it is irritating and may be mutagenic. Devices are being developed to remove some of these diesel particles from vehicle exhaust. A 70% reduction may soon be achieved in Europe.

In 1996, after a legal action launched by the American Lung Association, the EPA was forced to consider new air-quality standards for particulate matter. The proposed EPA limit on particulate emissions of less than 2.5 micrometers, a dimension that is about one-twentieth the diameter of a human hair, is no more than 20 to 65 micrograms of such particles per cubic meter of air. Some environmentalists would prefer a still tougher standard. Meeting these small particle standards will be very expensive and might not be possible. For example, dust reaching the United States from the Sahara Desert and salt in ocean spray are claimed to breach these new pollution standards. Particulate pollution in 25 out of 44 national parks is said to exceed the suggested standard. You can see the difficulties and expense in coping with this problem.

As you have seen, exposure to natural particles can cause illness, even death. An interesting, somewhat puzzling example is the relationship between thunder and lightning storms in London and a deluge of asthma attacks. A severe thunderstorm in London in June, 1994, was associated with 640 asthmatics swamping 12 emergency rooms, almost 10 times the usual, statistical number. These attacks were speculated to result from the stirring up of accumulated grass pollen, even though such pollen grains are generally larger than 5 micrometers, which would make them too large to enter the smallest air passages. It was suggested that smaller particles were formed by the storm. Other types of particles are thought to cause asthma attacks: for example, soybean dust in Barcelona, castor bean dust in Toledo, Ohio, and cockroach droppings within apartments and houses.

Electromagnetic Fields
(Are Electric Blankets Dangerous?)

The public has become concerned over potential health effects of magnetic fields. This fear stemmed from studies in the 1970s suggesting a possible link between childhood leukemia and proximity to certain types of power lines or utility transformers. There have also been hints of increased risk of breast cancer in adults exposed to high magnetic fields. A 1996 report issued by the National Academy of Sciences concluded that although electromagnetic fields (EMFs) appear capable of affecting biological tissues, their link to cancer is unproved.

As mentioned in the Overture, cellular phones produce EMFs. In 1993, on the television show, *Larry King Live*, a man claimed that a cellular phone caused his wife's brain tumor. This broadcast prompted lawsuits from other cellular phone users making similar claims. The manufacturers responded by sponsoring independent safety studies, which have not yet linked cellular phone use to cancer.

In Britain, a thorough study conducted in 2000 listed evidence indicating that cellular phone emissions can induce biological changes, but the health significance of these results is open to interpretation. Another article published in 2000 found that the type of microwave radiation emitted by older, analog cellular phones triggered a stress-response gene in roundworms; the same gene is found in people. These older devices emit signals at higher power levels and in a different pattern than newer digital phones do. Although it is not possible to prove that EMFs are safe, their greatest hazard is associated with traffic accidents related to the use of cellular phones while driving!

Magnetic fields are claimed to elicit their biological effects by acting on hormones. Some evidence suggests a possible mechanism by which EMFs might trigger cancer. This hypothesis is the so-called melatonin hypothesis, which claims that EMFs can perturb the body's natural concentrations of the brain hormone melatonin. This hormone is thought to be a natural suppressor of breast cancer cell growth. Some advocates claim that EMFs may also suppress the immune system. It is claimed that EMFs can alter two other hormones that affect cancer risk, estrogen and testosterone. Tests showed that laboratory rats exposed to 1,000-mG (milligauss) magnetic fields developed 50% more tumors than unexposed rats did. For comparison, simple household appliances deliver weaker fields. A hair dryer or vacuum cleaner at a distance of 6 inches produces only 700 mG. Other experiments indicate that intermittent fields, such as those from power surges, may pose more significant hazards than larger steady fields do. These surges pack a large amount of energy in a short period and occur when motors such as compressors in refrigerators or air-conditioners turn on. This issue is not settled, but it bears watching!

Some nonscientists believe that magnetic fields are healthful! Many individuals wear magnets as bracelets to ward off or relieve arthritis. I have met some physicians' wives who wear magnets for this reason, even though there is no scientific evidence that this practice is efficacious. Also, the retired famous tennis player Jimmy Connors wears magnetic inserts in his shoes. Perhaps a placebo effect is at work? A study reported in the *Journal of the American Medical Association* found no health difference between patients using real magnets and those using fake ones given as a placebo. Under certain circumstances, magnets can be dangerous because they can temporarily shut off pacemakers or defibrillators. More than 2 million Americans have implanted pacemakers, and 250,000 have defibrillators to help their hearts beat properly. Most therapeutic magnets never get close enough to the heart to affect a pacemaker; for safety, they should be kept six inches from the patient's chest. Magnet-laced mattress pads, neck braces, and shoulder wraps might be dangerous to individuals using these heart aids.

Sunlight

In the 1920s, daily therapeutic exposure to the sun—heliotherapy—was all the rage. Sunlight was touted as a cure for everything from acne to tuberculosis. By the 1940s, suntan lotions were being marketed, and a suntan became a symbol of health, wealth, and style. In the 1960s, sunlamps and tanning parlors grew popular. Later, it became evident that these parlors should be called melanoma centers because of sunlight's ability to induce skin cancer. The problem is a dangerous, invisible portion of the sunlight. Ultraviolet (UV) light is

Dust, Magnets, and Scuba Diving

a very energetic form of light; it contains enough energy to break chemical bonds and damage the molecules in your skin—even though you cannot see it. Bright sunlight contains different kinds of ultraviolet radiation—UVA and UVB radiation. It is easy to remember that UVB radiation causes burning and may initiate skin cancer, and UVA is linked with aging. Protecting yourself from both kinds of UV radiation is important. This energetic, invisible form of sunlight is strongest between 11 am and 3 pm on bright days. One way to estimate the intensity of UV light on a sunny day is to look at the length of your shadow; if you cannot see your shadow at all, UV light is intense. If your shadow is shorter than you are, you are still in a danger zone. If your shadow is quite long, you are less exposed to UVB rays, but UVA radiation remains in effect—all day. Furthermore, UV light is reflected off surfaces: water, sand, metal, and glass. Even when you are in the shade, UV light can reach you by reflection. The sun's rays can bounce off a stainless-steel table, an aluminum canoe, or water to penetrate the deeper layers of your skin.

There is more UV radiation at higher altitudes—for example, in the mountains. That is one reason you can get sunburned more rapidly at higher elevations. Snow reflects both UV and visible light, so skiers are particularly at risk for sunburn. While skiing in the mountains or lying on a bright beach, be certain your sunglasses are specified to remove UV as well as some of the visible light; otherwise, your eyes can become damaged, and you will not notice in time. Remember, you cannot see UV light, and therefore you do not sense the danger. UV rays can cause cataracts and damage to the retina.

Another nasty manifestation of exposure to the sun—especially the UV rays—is the delayed development of "cold sores," or fever blisters, on your lips. This effect is the result of the activation by UV light of a herpes simplex virus (related to the virus that causes genital herpes). Susceptible individuals carry the former virus for life! Upon each exposure to strong UV light, after a day or two, the cold sores reappear.

Sun protection is very important for babies, young children, and teenagers; two-thirds of most people's lifetime sun damage is incurred before the 15th birthday. Use of protective clothing made from a tightly woven fabric and a hat that shades the face, neck, and ears is very effective for preventing sunburn. When snorkeling in the tropics, wear a simple white T-shirt, which shields your back from the bright sun. Broad-spectrum sunscreen lotions offer some protection; dermatologists recommend those with a rating of at least SPF (sun-protection factor) 15. Do not be fooled by sunscreens of SPF 30; they give you only 3% more protection than one with SPF 15! Your lips are especially sensitive to damage because they are vulnerable to skin cancers. Use of these sunscreens gives you a false sense of security; they are not total blocks because they still allow some UV radiation through. Total blockout of sunlight is possible with a paste of a white compound, zinc oxide. This substance reflects visible light (that is why it appears white), but zinc oxide also reflects UV light, thus giving the wearer maximum protection. (Some formulations now come in colors.) Individuals who burn easily or carry the cold-sore virus are advised to use zinc oxide block-out cream.

Sunscreens not only fail to give you full protection against UV light, but they are not healthful for other reasons. Those lotions with a sun-protection factor above 8 block the UV wavelengths that convert precursors of vitamin D into the form needed by the body. It is further interesting that people who live in the northern parts of the United States, above the latitude of New York City, for example, do not produce enough vitamin D during the winter because the sun's rays are too weak.

The best protection from the sun is to have naturally black or very dark skin, but of course you have no control over this. Melanin is a natural skin pigment that protects individuals against the damage caused by sunlight. The less of it you have, the more careful you must be in the sun. A suntan generates some melanin but is not considered to protect you against skin cancer. If you have a Mediterranean skin that tans easily, you can still get skin cancer. If you have black skin, however, you may not be susceptible to skin cancer.

For those who get a malignant melanoma (skin cancer) and detect it early, the disease is usually curable by early surgical removal. But if the condition is ignored—or goes undiscovered—it can be fatal! Do you know of any deeply tanned dermatologists? I doubt it; that would be an oxymoron.

Chemical photosensitivity

There is another reason to be careful in the sun—certain drugs and some chemicals in suntan lotions can cause severe skin reactions with sun exposure. Chemicals that produce an adverse reaction with exposure to UV light are called photoreactive agents. These include both synthetic drugs and natural herbal remedies. Widely used medications containing photoreactive agents include antihistamines, used in cold and allergy medicines; nonsteroidal antiinflammatory drugs (NSAIDs), used to control pain and inflammation in arthritis; and antibiotics, including the tetracyclines and sulfa drugs. Herbal medicines such as the widely used antidepressant, St. John's Wort, can also be photosensitizers. Sunscreens containing bergamot oil, sandalwood oil, benzophenones, PABA, salicylates, anthranilates, and oxybenzone can all cause photosensitivity disorders. Many of these compounds are activated by the less energetic light, UVA radiation. These photosensitizers induce chemical changes that increase a person's sensitivity to light, causing the person to become photosensitized. Acute effects from short-term exposure include exaggerated sunburn conditions, eye burn, mild allergic reactions, hives, and eczema-like rashes with itching, swelling, blistering, oozing, and scaling of the skin. Chronic effects from long-term exposure include premature skin aging, stronger allergic reactions, cataracts, blood vessel damage, a weakened immune system, and skin cancer!

Some medications cause photoallergic reactions, in which UV light structurally changes the drug, causing formation of antibodies that result in an allergic reaction. This effect can occur immediately after exposure to the sun or may be delayed for up to 3 months. Synthetic medicines, such as the over-the-counter pain-relievers containing ibuprofen, as well as natural cosmetics that contain musk ambrette, sandalwood oil, and bergamot oil have been reported to produce photoallergic reactions. The degree of photosensitivity varies among individuals. People with fair skin are the most susceptible, but it is not uncommon for dark-skinned individuals to have chronic photodermatitis. Whether or not the use of sunscreens helps protect against photosensitivity is not clear.

In rare cases, people can become photosensitized from some food they eat. Perhaps you remember that plants such as parsnips and celery produce natural so-called phytochemicals on their surfaces that can absorb UV light and thereby become very reactive. These photoactive substances can act as carcinogens or mutagens because they damage DNA. These potentially dangerous phytochemicals are called furanocoumarins. For the vast majority of people consuming a typical Western-style diet, ingestion of the photoactive furanocoumarins is generally low, and toxicity as a consequence of their ingestion is relatively rare. The human body has liver enzymes that detoxify these substances before they can become activated by sunlight and cause harm. There are exceptions. In one report, a woman consumed a pound of celery root, drank the water it was prepared in, and then an hour later went to a tanning salon, where she received a massive exposure to ultraviolet light. She suffered severe skin damage from photosensitization.

Inherited photosensitivity

Some unfortunate individuals have an inherited photosensitivity; they cannot make the iron-containing part of hemoglobin, the molecule on red blood cells that carries oxygen. Those who are afflicted with these congenital disorders, about 1 out of 25,000 people, should avoid exposure to the sun, which can result in dark blotches on the person's exposed skin. This family of diseases, called porphyrias, has many symptoms, including mental illness and skin lesions that are aggravated by sunlight. Porphyrias have a long history; legends about vampires and werewolves may have grown out of porphyrias. Perhaps you recall the 1995 movie *The Madness of King George,* which was based on King George III's mental disorder—a result of porphyria. George was the British monarch who lost the American colonies.

Underwater Dangers (Scuba Diving)

Scuba diving in clear tropical waters teeming with brightly colored fish is exhilarating. Equipment for diving under the sea is relatively inexpensive and easy to rent, and instruction is readily available in seaside resorts. Be careful, though; scuba diving is a potentially dangerous activity! Why? What is the underlying science? Amateur divers need to understand the behavior of gases, especially the solubility of gases in their blood and body fluids. Divers breathe compressed air. As a diver descends through the water, he or she is subject to the pressure at the surface *plus* the pressure of a water column proportional to the diver's depth. Table 9 shows the pressure in atmospheres at different depths of seawater (which is slightly more dense than fresh water). The pressure of the air divers breathe (through a "scuba" regulator) must be equal to the total surrounding pressure. Deeper dives therefore require a diver to breathe air at even higher pressure. This sport can have several serious consequences if mistakes are made.

Dust, Magnets, and Scuba Diving

Table 9   Increase in pressure with increase of depth in water[a]

Pressure (atmospheres)	Depth (feet)
1	surface
2	33
3	66
4	99
5	132
6	165
10	297

[a]Adapted from: Ecuyer, A. 1968. *The New Science of Skin and Scuba Diving.* New York: Association Press.

The human lung is not very expandable; it is like a fragile balloon. Divers must continuously exhale and take care never to hold their breath when ascending. Otherwise, the air pressure in their lungs would become greater than the surrounding pressure in the body—in which case the lungs might rupture! Even when 5 feet deep in a pool, a diver taking in air from a regulator, and then holding his or her breath while abruptly ascending to the surface, risks serious injury because of the lower pressure at the water surface; the air in the lung expands, but the lung does not. This response is illustrated in Figure 22.

At greater depths, other dangers arise. It is important to realize that the amount of any gas that will dissolve in a liquid depends on the pressure of that gas. In a mixture of gases, each different gas has its own "partial pressure," which corresponds to the pressure of the fraction of that individual gas in the overall gas mixture. An example of mixed gases would be the principal gases in air: nitrogen and oxygen. If the partial pressure of nitrogen in the compressed air from the scuba tank becomes high enough, a diver can become intoxicated by the additional nitrogen that dissolves in his or her blood.

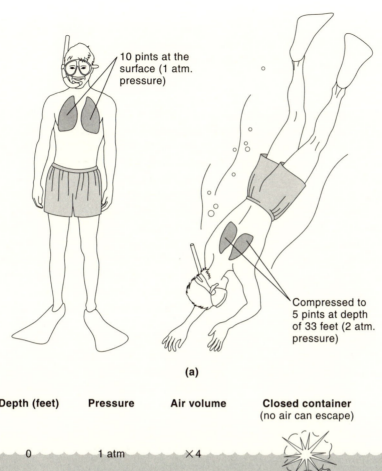

10 pints at the surface (1 atm. pressure)

Compressed to 5 pints at depth of 33 feet (2 atm. pressure)

(a)

Depth (feet)	Pressure	Air volume	Closed container (no air can escape)
0	1 atm	×4	
33	2 atm	×2	
66	3 atm	×1⅓	
99	4 atm	×1	Air

(b)

Figure 22. Effect of pressure on the lungs. **A.** Lungs' volume decreases twofold at a 33-foot depth in water. **B.** If you hold your breath, blocking the airway to your lungs while you ascend, your lungs will overexpand much like the sealed bag.

Dust, Magnets, and Scuba Diving

The famous French oceanographer Jacques Cousteau called this effect the "rapture of the depths." Every 50 feet of depth is equivalent to drinking another dry martini; like alcohol intoxication, susceptibility to nitrogen intoxication varies with the individual. Deep diving, below 100 feet, becomes more dangerous—rarely can even experienced divers go deeper than 200 feet by breathing compressed air. This narcotic effect is not well understood, but it clearly involves an increased amount of dissolved nitrogen in the blood, which becomes more concentrated as the partial pressure of nitrogen is increased. Helium has a lesser narcotic effect than nitrogen. For this reason, mixtures of helium and oxygen are used by professional divers for deep dives, but these mixtures pose additional problems. For example, excessive oxygen is toxic! At oxygen partial pressure greater than 1.5 to 1.7 atmospheres, oxygen poisoning effects can cause convulsions. Deep-sea scuba divers use tanks filled with dilute oxygen in helium so that, at great depths, they do not take in too much oxygen. This toxic effect of oxygen must also be taken into account during certain medical procedures in which patients are treated with oxygen-enriched air, for example, to accelerate healing of stress fractures.

Another serious concern for deep-sea divers is the decompression illness referred to as "the bends." This disease has been known for many years. In the 1870s, for example, 119 builders who were working under pressure in tunnels while constructing the St. Louis Bridge experienced decompression illness. Of the 119 workers who became ill, 14 died. This malady can also occur among astronauts who don low-pressure space suits, as well as professional and amateur scuba divers. Tissue and blood supersaturated with dissolved gas can form gas bubbles if the pressure is abruptly reduced upon reaching the surface. After exposure to higher pressures of a gas, bubbles form as the external gas pressure is decreased in much the same way as opening a pop bottle that is under pressure—the gas dissolved in the soda comes out as bubbles. In people with decompression illness, this condition (paralysis, shock, weakness, dizziness, numbness, difficulty breathing, and limb pain) results from the formation of gas bubbles in the central nervous system (the brain and the spinal cord). Researchers have found bubbles in the blood streams of divers and also of aviators subject to sudden decompression of only 0.3 atmosphere. The effects of this condition may show up several hours or even days after exposure to compressed gas. For this reason, it is dangerous to fly or even drive through the mountains too soon after a deep-water scuba dive. After ascending from the depths, a diver may need to decompress at intermediate depths, or if signs of serious illness arise, treatment in a hyperbaric decompression chamber may be necessary.

About 10% of the population is in even greater danger of contracting decompression disease because of an abnormal heart condition (a patent foramen ovale). Such people are five times more likely to suffer decompression problems than are those without this condition.

Considering these dangers, you can understand why scuba divers in the United States are required to take lessons and become certified. However, a new kind of assisted diving, called "snuba," so far does not require a license. Snuba divers receive compressed air through a tube from an overhead boat and descend to depths up to 20 feet. Do you think the lack of certification for this type of diving is wise? Recall the danger of scuba diving in only 5 feet of water.

Deep-diving animals such as whales and penguins go much deeper for longer periods and yet show no signs of the bends or other ills that plague human divers. For example, the deepest-diving air-breather is the sperm whale, which has been tracked to depths of 1.2 miles and is thought capable of diving even deeper. How do these deep-diving animals manage such feats without getting the bends? The answer is still somewhat of a mystery, but there are some hints. These creatures have much higher stores of the oxygen-storing pigment myoglobin in their tissues than land mammals do. Their heartbeats fall to very low rates—as few as three beats a minute—and the lungs of some deep divers such as penguins and seals are thought to collapse under the high pressures found at great depths. Their temperatures may also fall, indicating a metabolic slowdown. Nevertheless, why they do not experience decompression illness is not clear.

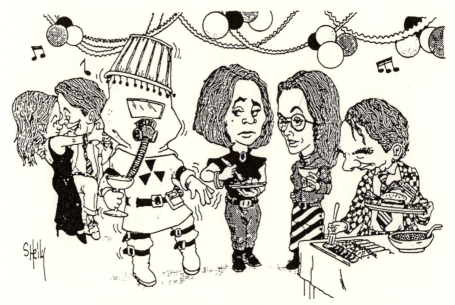

"HE'S THE HALF-LIFE OF THE PARTY"

CHAPTER

CHAPTER

10

We Are All Radioactive!

RADIATION HAZARDS are often discussed in the media, but this subject is poorly understood by the general public. This topic has become fertile ground for scientific demagoguery. Some communities have even passed laws to create a so-called "nuclear-free environment" (implying radiation-free) within their boundaries. This is quite impossible; as you will learn, we are all radioactive. Your body emits 6,000 gamma rays per minute! In fact, as you read this book, you are radiating your near neighbors! Beyond that, we are constantly being exposed to radiation from the Earth and the sky. On the other hand, I do not want to leave you with the impression that excess radiation is not dangerous. As with toxic substances, the degree of danger depends on the type, amount, and location of the radiation you receive.

I will start by defining radiation. In this case, I am *not* referring to radiowaves or microwaves or to infrared, visible, or even ultraviolet radiation. The individual photons of these forms of electromagnetic radiation have insufficient energy to knock an electron out of a molecule, thus ionizing it and forming a free radical (a very reactive molecule with an unpaired electron). Here, what I am referring to is ionizing radiation, which encompasses X-rays, gamma rays, and atomic particles (Figure 23). The photons and particles in ionizing radiation do have sufficient energy to remove electrons from molecules.

Whereas nonionizing radiation is relatively harmless, ionizing radiation can have a destructive effect on living tissue. Ionizing radiation is associated with radioactivity. High-energy radiation was discovered in 1885, when Wilhelm Roentgen observed a previously unknown, penetrating radiation, which he called X-rays. This was followed by Madame Curie's discovery in 1898 of the radioactive elements polonium and radium. These heavy elements fall in that part

209

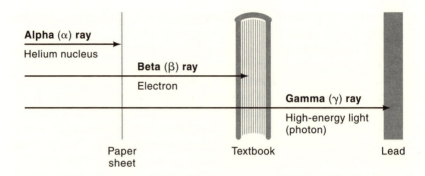

Figure 24. The penetrating power of three types of ionizing radiation, alpha, beta, and gamma (concept by Mark Hart).

Using a hand-held Geiger counter, a device used to measure small amounts of radiation, you can find radioactive items in antique stores. These pieces of uranium glassware can also be detected by using an ultraviolet lamp (black light), which causes these items to glow (fluoresce) in the dark. A company in Ohio still makes green juice glasses, butter dishes, and figurines out of glass containing uranium. These objects give off both alpha and beta rays, which pose no danger because alpha rays do not escape the glass, and the beta rays barely penetrate your body.

Many items once contained radioactive components but these are no longer manufactured because they are possibly hazardous. Smoke detectors once contained radium; dentures were made from thorium; luminous clock and watch dials used radium; and some paint pigments contained uranium oxides. In fact, some radium-dial painters got cancer of the mouth by licking the ends of their paint brushes! These and many other radioactive items have been discontinued, although a few remain in use today. One example is an old-model heart pacemaker containing plutonium-238, which is still in some people!

Other radioactive materials still in common use in this country and abroad include the following. Battery-operated smoke detectors usually contain americium-241. The ultra-high-quality lenses in some Pentax cameras use thorium glass. The emergency exit signs in some commercial aircraft and movie theaters as well as airport-runway night lights use tritium (a beta emitter—tritium is the second

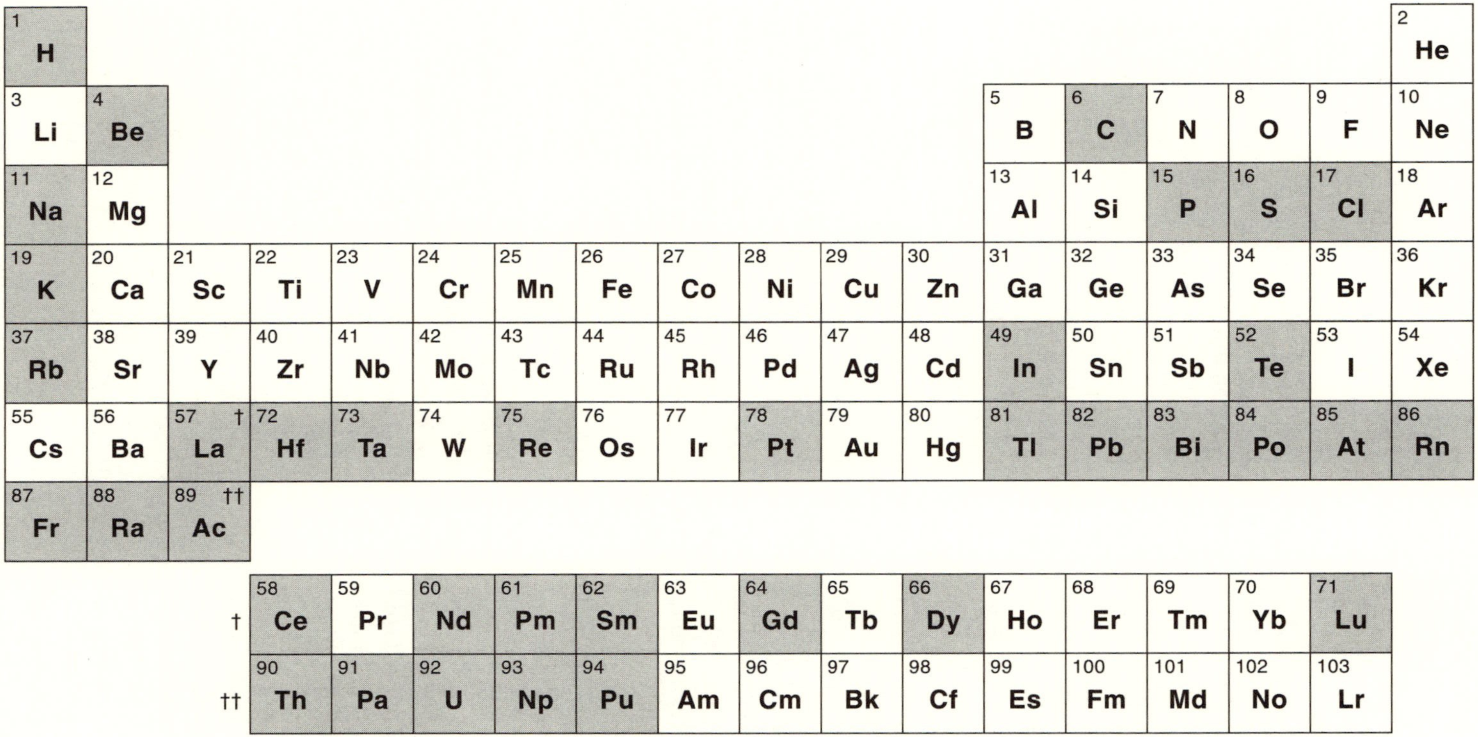

Figure 25. Darkened quadrants correspond to elements that have naturally occurring radioactive isotopes.

213

heavy-isotope of hydrogen, the one used to make hydrogen bombs). The British military and police have been using tritium-powered flashlights, which last up to 20 years! Many propane gas lanterns use radioactive thorium oxide in the mantle. Some modern lightning rods also contain polonium at the rod tip. None of these items is regarded as dangerous.

The high density of uranium metal has many modern uses. Did you know that a Boeing 747 aircraft has 3,000 pounds of uranium in its control surfaces as a counterweight? Some sailboats use uranium as a ballast. Uranium metal is also used to clad military tanks, especially in Russia and the United States. This uranium is depleted of the isotope used to make atomic bombs, but it is still radioactive.

Elementary particles are also used to detect dangerous substances. For instance, neutron beams are used to search for high-energy explosives in airline luggage. You probably know that some radioisotopes are used in medicine. For example, the following ones are used as tracers in diagnostic testing: ^{18}F, fluorine-18 (brain); ^{99}Tc, technetium-99 (heart, thyroid, liver, and lungs); ^{131}I, iodine-131 (thyroid); ^{201}Tl, thallium-201 (heart muscle); and ^{11}C, carbon-11 (general metabolism). Each gives off some form of ionizing radiation that can be easily detected. Keep in mind that in higher concentrations, these radioactive isotopes are dangerous, but not at the doses used in diagnosis.

High-energy ionizing radiation is used for cancer radiation therapy. A well-known example, cobalt-60 (^{60}Co), a gamma emitter, is used to treat brain tumors. Again, larger doses of this radiation applied to the whole body could be lethal. These radiation treatments are usually focused on the site of the tumor. Cancer cells, which grow rapidly, are more susceptible to damage by radiation than most normal body cells, but certain fast-growing normal body tissues are also susceptible to damage. A well-known side effect of radiation treatment is the loss of hair. Hair growth is comparatively rapid, and therefore hair cells are more susceptible to radiation damage. After the treatment is stopped, the hair grows back.

X-rays were once widely used not only for diagnosis but to treat all sorts of ailments. Because of the possible danger of accumulated doses, however, diagnostic X-ray doses are now about 40 times lower than they once were. Other measurements and treatments with X-rays were discontinued after their potential danger was realized. Two examples of such discontinued practices are hair removal and shoe sizing. Another use of ionizing radiation is to sterilize insects such as male fruit flies to control infestations. No one yet seems to object to this practice, but we may not have heard the last word from extreme animal-rights activists!

The public's fear of radiation is based partly on their belief that radiation is a substance, rather than a form of energy. An example of this misconception appeared in a San Francisco newspaper article reporting the objections of neighbors to the construction of a crematorium near their property. They argued that many of the people being turned into ashes had been receiving radiation treatment for cancer and would therefore emit radiation when they were cremated. The newspaper reporter writing the story promulgated this misinformation because of his own scientific ignorance. Radiation is just energy, not a substance. As you will see below, ionizing radiation is everywhere!

Radiation in Nature

We are constantly being bombarded by natural radiation from cosmic rays and from naturally occurring radioisotopes. These natural sources are shown in Figure 26, along with additional sources.

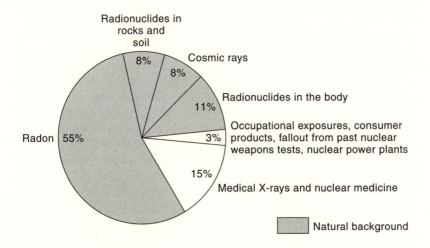

Figure 26. Comparisons between radiation exposure of an average person in the U.S. from natural and anthropogenic sources. Actual dosages may vary widely.

Cosmic radiation from outer space is blocked to some extent by the Earth's atmosphere; your exposure to this radiation depends on where you live and how often you fly. For example, your exposure in Denver, the mile-high city, is approximately twice that of someone in Washington, D.C. In a plane at 30,000 feet, your exposure is approximately 0.5 mrem (about 1/20 of one cent's worth; remember m stands for milli, or 1/1000). However, while flying in a supersonic jet in the presence of a giant solar flare, your exposure range is $1 to $10 per hour. Remember that the yearly limit mandated by the US government for a nuclear plant worker is 5 rem, or $5 worth. In fact, during solar flares, air controllers reroute the Concord supersonic jet so as to minimize the exposure of passengers and crew to cosmic radiation. Astronauts spending three months in the Skylab receive the equivalent of $7.50. The typical commercial airline pilot gets only about $1 per year.

Some natural radiation from within the Earth comes from uranium, thorium, and their "daughter" isotopes formed by radioactive decay. In several locations around the country, radioactive radon gas seeps out of the ground and is also found in some well water. Many individuals are subject to some radiation exposure from building materials such as rock, stone, and concrete. For example, Grand Central Station in New York City and St. Peter's Square in Rome emit about 50¢ a year's worth—not much, but something. Other radiation released into the environment comes from sources such as burning coal. According to the EPA, 616 million tons of coal were burned in the United States in 1982. This practice released the equivalent of 801 tons of uranium and 1971 tons of thorium! Most estimates put the number of deaths in the United States at 10,000 per year from cancer and respiratory diseases caused by burning coal, but only part of this death rate is the result of radioactivity. Interestingly, nuclear power plants expose the populace to much less radiation than coal-burning does. The real danger posed by nuclear reactors stems from their potential for large-scale disaster, which is always present. Accidents at Three Mile Island in Pennsylvania in March, 1979, and at Chernobyl, Ukraine, in April, 1986, are reminders of this sleeping tiger. The former killed or injured no one, but the latter certainly did. In the United States and western Europe, secondhand cigarette smoke is a greater health risk than the proximity of a nuclear power plant. No study has ever found an increase in childhood leukemia or any other cancers among people living close to properly operating nuclear power plants in the United States or other countries.

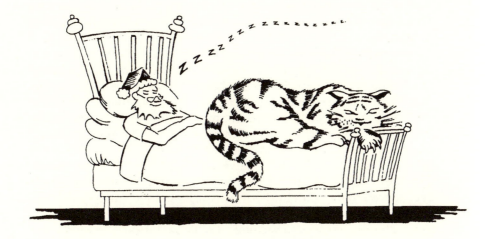

Nuclear Power: a sleeping tiger......"

One other large but little-recognized source of radiation pollution is *cat litter*! A major component of most cat litter is bentonite clay, which naturally contains uranium and thorium in trace amounts. Eventually this litter is dumped into landfills throughout the country. Each year, about 23,000 pounds of uranium and 57,000 pounds of thorium from cat litter are thus put into the ground, eventually to be leached out into the nation's groundwater.

You, yourself, are radioactive! If you submit to a whole-body scan with a sensitive radiometer, it will easily record the radiation you are emitting. This emission comes largely from minuscule amounts of the radioactive potassium isotope ^{40}K, which is found throughout nature in food and in our bodies. Remember that potassium and carbon are essential to life. We also ingest some uranium, which is present in tiny amounts in most of the food we eat. Estimates are that we each eat about 1.3 micrograms of uranium each day. One can calculate that this amounts to ingestion of about 10^{15} (a million-billion) atoms of uranium daily. An average human body experiences about 500,000 radioactive disintegrations per minute. Your body emits approximately 6,000 gamma rays per minute; because these gamma rays are very penetrating, you are irradiating your neighbors!

Some people would say that because it is natural, the radioactive potassium in your body must be less hazardous than radiation from the infamous synthetic isotope, cobalt-60 (^{60}Co). In fact, the gamma rays from postassium-40 (^{40}K) are more energetic than those from ^{60}Co (1.46 versus 1.33 million electron volts, MeV). For comparison, about 4 electron volts is an amount equivalent to the energy holding two carbon atoms together in organic molecules.

The important difference between ^{40}K and ^{60}Co is not the amount of energy in each gamma ray photon but rather the number of gamma ray photons that assault the body over a given time. Think of a 50-caliber, single-shot rifle versus a whole bank of 30-caliber machine guns. The rate or speed of a chemical process may be expressed by its half-life, the amount of time required for one-half of a reaction, in this case nuclear decay, to occur. Cobalt-60 has a half-life of 5.27 years, whereas potassium-40 has a much longer half-life of 1.25 billion years! This means that cobalt-60 decays at a much faster rate than potassium-40 does. During the time that a single potassium-40 nucleus decays, giving off one gamma ray, 2.4 billion cobalt-60 nuclei have decayed, each one giving off one gamma ray! If we were to calculate the masses of the two different radioisotopes needed to give off an equivalent amount of radiation, we would find that 1 microgram of ^{60}Co (much less than a grain of salt) would emit the same number of gamma rays as 6 pounds of isotopically pure ^{40}K. It is also important to remember that potassium-40 is a minor isotope, which means there is only a very tiny amount of the radioactive potassium-40 present in the ordinary, nonradioactive potassium-39. Thus, 27 tons of ordinary potassium (a cube with 10 feet per side) would be required to equal the radioactivity of 1 microgram of ^{60}Co! These figures should remind you of the tremendous range of numbers that arise from dealing with atoms, rates of transformations, and ultrasensitive analytical methods.

An incident at the Los Alamos National Laboratory in New Mexico illustrates the fear that even experts can develop over natural radioactivity. Some technicians were scanning various rooms of the metallurgical research building looking for any radioactive contamination. They discovered a strong signal from their instruments in the lunch and conference room, whereupon they evacuated the entire building on a radiation alert. Later, they found the culprit to be a box of "no-salt," which is a potassium chloride salt substitute. The small amount of naturally occurring potassium-40 was giving off gamma rays, as it does in your body. There was no danger, just a sensitive measuring device.

Radioactive elements with short half-lives (meaning they decompose rapidly) are said to be "hot" and are usually more dangerous. On the other hand, an element with a very long half-life will necessarily be in the environment for a very long time. Plutonium, an artificial element, is an example; ^{239}Pu has a half-life of 24,000 years. If sufficiently large quantities of long-lived radioisotopes enter and remain in your body, they can be dangerous.

The major risks associated with radioactive elements depend not only on their rates of decomposition, but also on whether we ingest these substances and how long they remain in our body. An alpha-particle emitter presents only a minor hazard when outside the body because the alpha particles collide with molecules in the air and are stopped before they have a chance to enter the skin. On the other hand, if an alpha emitter is inhaled or ingested, it can create serious problems in the tissue in which it concentrates. Under these circumstances, alpha emitters are more dangerous per decay event than are beta or even the powerful gamma emitters. Apparently, these localized alpha particles are better absorbed in sensitive tissue.

Plutonium is the radioactive metallic element named for the planet Pluto. Although it exists in minute quantities in nature, plutonium is the creation of the World War II Manhattan Project to design the first nuclear weapons and the subsequent arms race. At the end of the Cold War, the world was left with several hundred tons of this toxic element; its disposal is a major societal problem. Unlike rotten eggs, plutonium cannot be thrown away without major consequences.

Unfortunately, plutonium cannot currently be employed to generate atomic power, as plutonium reactors are not yet economical. The possibility of terrorist diversion, theft, and illicit sales makes the disposal of plutonium a pressing, worldwide problem. The weapons-grade isotope, plutonium-239, has a half-life of 24,000 years, is hazardous, and should be kept out of the biosphere. What about the toxicity of plutonium? It is sometimes described as an exceedingly toxic substance and has been claimed by some environmental activists to be the most toxic substance known. Actually, plutonium is relatively harmless unless you eat or inhale it. The principal radiation from a nearby plutonium sample is blocked by your clothing, but within your body, plutonium is taken up in your bones and remains there to radiate over many years. Plutonium's risks to human health depend on its form. Inhalation is more dangerous than ingestion. Risks to health depend upon the method of exposure, the isotope, the particle size, and its chemical form.

The weapons isotope, plutonium-239, is weakly radioactive; it emits primarily alpha particles (helium nuclei), which do not even penetrate paper or human skin. The other radiation (neutrons and weak gamma rays) can penetrate the body, but large amounts of plutonium would be needed to form serious radiation doses. Another isotope, plutonium-241, forms americium-241, which poses a greater radiation danger because it is a stronger gamma emitter.

Once inside the body, plutonium is highly toxic. Upon exposure to air, plutonium metal oxidizes to form plutonium oxide (PuO_2); this powdery substance can lodge in the lungs, where it has a biological half-life of about 500 days; alpha particles from this oxide can cause cancer. Small quantities of inhaled plutonium oxide can be transported by the lymphocytes into the bloodstream and end up in bone or liver. If weakly soluble plutonium oxide dissolves in water, ingestion of only a few millionths of a gram can cause cancer after prolonged periods. Surprisingly little data exist on the human-health effects of plutonium. Epidemiologic data are scarce and probably have been kept secret.

The worst plutonium polluter in the United States was the Rocky Flats plant in Colorado, where purified plutonium metal was milled and shaped into bomb cores. The plutonium wastes from this plant have been packed into barrels and are awaiting future burial in a salt mine in New Mexico, if that repository is ever permitted to open. Building 771 at Rocky Flats was recently judged as the most hazardous plutonium site in the country; the air ducts are thought to contain enough material to make seven atomic bombs. Wind-blown dust from this site, exacerbated by two fires at the plant, has contaminated the outskirts of Denver. Because acute poisoning or any immediate harm from plutonium has not been documented in human beings, we must await epidemiologic studies of the exposed people in the downwind population of Denver before this problem can be evaluated.

We Are All Radioactive!

You would imagine the Japanese would be very sensitive to the hazards of plutonium. Surprisingly, the Japanese-owned Power Reactor and Nuclear Fuel Development Corporation has distributed a video that portrays plutonium as harmless! Apparently, this video was designed to reassure people living near a new plutonium–uranium breeder reactor of their safety. Such reactors produce more usable nuclear fuel than they consume.

Radium, whose chemistry resembles that of calcium, is taken up by the skeleton, and for this reason radium is especially dangerous. Nobel Prize–winner Marie Curie seems to have died of the effects of exposure to radium, even though throughout her life she tended to deny the perils of radiation. Her daughter, Irene Joliot-Curie, and son-in-law, Frederic Joliot—also Nobel Prize winners—both died of diseases induced by radiation.

Other radioactive isotopes, such as strontium-90 and iodine-131, are also particularly dangerous because they collect and remain in specific parts of your body, such as the bone marrow. On the other hand, we do inhale radioactive radon gas. Because it is an inert gas, you might think radon would soon leave the body. Unfortunately, atoms of polonium-218, a radioactive decay product of radon, attach to fine aerosol particles that can stick to the inner walls of the lung. There, a series of nuclear decay events emit both gamma radiation and alpha particles, which can result in lung cancer. Smokers are especially susceptible to this hazard.

To understand the possible danger from ionizing radiation, it is important to consider three models that have been used to predict biological response to various doses of ionizing radiation. These three theories are plotted in Figure 27. The first theory (the hormesis model) is that low doses of radiation are *beneficial,* whereas high doses are harmful. The second theory (the threshold theory) proposes that there is a threshold level above which the radiation becomes harmful. The third model (the linear theory) predicts that all radiation is harmful, no matter how low the dose. The hormesis model predicts that high and low doses produce opposite effects. This hypothesis is based on the results of many experimental animal studies that demonstrate longer survival rates upon exposure of a subject to low doses of radiation. The data supporting this hormesis theory have been developed over many years in different laboratories. Even so, people have a hard time believing that low doses of ionizing radiation could be beneficial. Remember that the body takes many

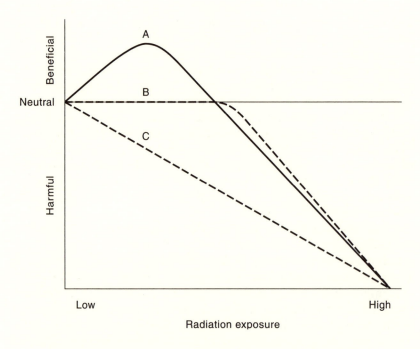

Figure 27. Three models of the biological response to radiation:
A, hormesis; **B**, threshold; **C**, linear.

"hits" from reactive oxygen species formed as byproducts during respiration and that DNA has built-in mechanisms of proofreading and damage repair. Mammalian cells on average undergo about 10,000 DNA modification events per cell per hour. Studies using X-rays show that a large, instantaneous dose is fatal, whereas the same dose spread over a period of time is not. The no-threshold danger level in the first theory seems unreasonable in light of the presence of background radiation and the constant bombardment all living systems experience from reactive oxygen species as a result of radiation. This subject remains controversial, but some scientists believe the public has been needlessly frightened and deceived, and hundreds of billions of dollars have been wasted protecting us from low levels of ionizing radiation. Moreover, radiation can be useful in protecting the public from other health hazards.

We Are All Radioactive!

Irradiation of Food

Dangers from infectious biological agents can be remedied by employing ionizing radiation. One potentially dangerous substance or process can be used to mollify another dangerous agent. For example, gamma radiation from ^{60}Co can be used to kill bacteria in chicken and vegetables. Sealed packets of gamma-irradiated food may have a shelf-life of more than a year without refrigeration. However, the American public is largely afraid of this method because many people believe that the gamma rays are a substance and leave the food contaminated.

In 1999, the Food and Drug Administration approved the irradiation of red meat to reduce microbial contamination in food. The irradiation of ground beef was a response to estimates that as many as 9,000 deaths per year may be caused by bacterial contamination of food. Irradiation is the only known method of eliminating from raw meat the deadly *Escherichia coli* O157:H7, the bacterium responsible for several fatal food-poisoning incidents involving hamburgers. Irradiation also reduces contamination from *Listeria, Salmonella,* and *Campylobacter* species. Earlier, in 1986, the FDA approved the use of radiation to destroy insects and toxic mold in wheat, potatoes, fresh fruits, and spices. In 1990, it authorized the radiation of chicken to kill bacteria such as *Salmonella* or *Campylobacter,* which are the two biggest causes of food poisoning in the United States. Until 1997, the only foods actually treated this way were spices and exotic Hawaiian fruits like papaya, to kill fruitflies.

Many people fear ionizing radiation technology because of their belief that irradiation makes food radioactive. Irradiated food will not budge the meter on a Geiger counter, but the practice does stir up controversy on talk-shows. In truth, irradiation simply adds energy in amounts similar to cooking. The food keeps its taste, texture, and nutritional value without retaining any radiation. There is a slight loss of vitamins in some foods, but no more than by cooking. Radiation kills bacteria by fracturing their genetic material (DNA) so the bacteria cannot multiply. The shelf-life of irradiated red meat, such as hamburger or sausages, can be extended for about 10 days at a cost of three to six cents a pound.

The US government requires that labels specify when food has been irradiated. It is amusing that, to alleviate the public's fear, the

FDA will permit the words "treated by radiation" to appear in *smaller print*. This practice may be effective for those consumers who need reading glasses. Others advocate using the term "cold Pasteurization" to keep fears at bay. The radiation source used for food treatment is cobalt-60. Scientific studies conclude that irradiated food is safe. This controversy is an interesting concept in which a method feared by the nonscientific public may actually prevent illness and death among consumers. In 2000, the United States Department of Agriculture ruled that produce could not be labeled organic food if it had been irradiated.

There are 50 known strains of *E. coli* that, if ingested, can lead to bloody diarrhea, kidney failure, and death. In 1997, the USDA and other governmental agencies tested for only one variety, *E. coli* O157:H7, which had been associated with extensive foodborne disease, being a leading cause of kidney failure in children and an encephalitis-like disease in older people. This species has been found in as many as 1.5% to 5% of dairy cows, which have been nicknamed the Typhoid Marys of these bacterial epidemics because of their carrying this bacterium harmlessly in their feces. The *E. coli* O157:H7 strain is very dangerous, tough, and virulent. It can live in acidic environments such as unpasteurized apple cider and in the salty brine processing of venison jerky. The organism is armed with a nasty toxin thought to have originated in the bacterium *Shigella*. The gene coding for this toxin was probably transferred between the two bacterial species by a virus. Viruses that infect bacteria can sometimes pick up a gene from one bacterium and carry it to another. To avoid this nasty new bug, people are advised to eat only hamburger that has been cooked at 160° F or has been irradiated. Consumers should thoroughly wash produce and avoid unpasteurized apple juice and raw milk products. For gourmets who enjoy rare beef, irradiated hamburger might be a better choice, if they can overcome their fear of irradiation.

It has been suggested that irradiation of shellfish, at one-fourth the dose approved for fresh meat, can completely eliminate the dangerous microorganism *Vibrio vulnificus* from oysters. One special-interest group that has worked to prevent food irradiation from winning public acceptance has, at the same time, decried the health threat posed by oysters. This is a good example of the conflict that occurs in matters of science and public policy.

EPILOGUE

There Is No Free Lunch!

THINKING BACK OVER EXAMPLES in this book, you may appreciate the complexity of the science behind public-policy issues and realize that there are no simple solutions to toxicity, ecology, and public health problems. Many natural substances that are vital to life under some circumstances are dangerous under other circumstances. This book should help you realize that everything that is "natural" is not necessarily safe. Many public phobias are grounded in misinformation, misunderstanding, and in some instances, scientific demagoguery. For exposures to agents that may be dangerous, the amount, the type, and the time-course of exposure are all important in determining the extent of the risk. Risk—benefit analysis is essential, as most agents are neither 100% good or bad. I hope readers have learned that there is no "free lunch" in matters of toxic and dangerous substances. In summary, putting these risks in the context of potential dangers from other common human activities is instructive. To illustrate this point, Table 10 ranks 30 exposures in the order that they are most likely to contribute to death. These data show, for example, that pesticide exposure is more dangerous than taking prescription antibiotics, but less dangerous than the risks of using nuclear power or playing football!

Table 10   Ranking of 30 exposures contributing to deaths in the United States[a]

1. Smoking	16. Firefighting
2. Drinking alcohol	17. Police work
3. Motor vehicles	18. Contraceptives
4. Hand guns	19. Commercial aviation
5. Electric power	20. Nuclear power
6. Motorcycles	21. Mountain climbing
7. Swimming	22. Power machines
8. Surgery	23. American football
9. X-rays	24. Skiing
10. Railroads	25. Vaccinations
11. General aviation	26. Food coloring
12. Construction	27. Food preservation
13. Bicycles	28. Pesticides
14. Hunting	29. Prescription antibiotics
15. Home appliances	30. Spray cans

[a]From The Chemical Society. *Chemistry in Britain*, July 1998, p. 20.

Further Reading

Chapter 1

Ackerman, D. 1990. *A natural history of the senses.* New York: Chapman.

Bingham, S. 1987. *The everyman companion to food and nutrition.* London: J. M. Dent.

Braun, S. 1996. *Buzz: The science and lore of alcohol and caffeine.* New York: Oxford Univ. Press.

Coady, C. 1993. *Chocolate, the food of the gods.* London: Pavilion Books.

Davies, J., Dickerson, J. 1991. *Nutrient content of food portions.* London: Royal Society of Chemistry.

Diamandia, S. G. J., Eletherios, P., Goldberg, D. M. 1997. Wine as a biological fluid: History, production, and role in disease prevention. *Clin. Lab. Anal.* 11:287–313.

Emsley, J. 1998. *Molecules at an exhibition: The science of everyday life.* Oxford: Oxford Univ. Press.

Emsley, J. 1994. *The consumer's good chemical guide: A jargon-free guide to the chemicals of everyday life.* Oxford: W. H. Freeman.

Evans, D. 1998. Agrochemicals: Benefits and risks. *Chem. Br.* 34(7):20.

Fackelmann, K. 1997. The bitter truth: Do some people inherit a distaste for broccoli? *Science News* 152:24. (Discussion of supertasters.)

Fackelmann, K. 1997. Power failure: What happens when muscle cells run out of fuel. *Science News* 152:206.

Goldstein, D. B. 1983. *Pharmacology of alcohol.* New York: Oxford Univ. Press.

Hampl, J. S., Hampl, W. S. 1997. Pellagra and the origin of a myth: Evidence from European literature and folklore. *J. R. Soc. Med.* 90:636–638.

Harvard Medical School. 2000. Kidney stones. *Harvard Men's Health Watch* 4(9):1.

Harvard Medical School. 1999. High-tech dining: Is America ready? *Harvard Men's Health Watch* 4(3):1. (Genetic engineering, irradiated food.)

Harvard Medical School. 1998. Americans and red meat: A love–hate relationship. *Harvard Health Letter* 23(7):1.

Lison M., Blondheim, S. H., Melmed, R. N. 1980. A polymorphism of the
ability to smell urinary metabolites of asparagus. *Br. Med. J.* 218:1676.
Lucia, S. P. 1963. *A history of wine as therapy.* Philadelphia: Lippincott.
Mayo Clinic. 2000. Grapefruit juice influences certain cholesterol drugs.
Mayo Clinic Health Letter 18(3):4.
Mitchel, S. C., Waring, R. H., Land, D., Thorpe, W. V. 1987. Odorous urine
following asparagus ingestion in man. *Experientia* 43:382.
Moore, P. 1996. Fueled for life. *Inside Science,* 87:1; in *New Scientist*
149:2012. (Energy flow through plants and animals.)
Pond, C. M. 1998. *The fats of life.* Cambridge: Cambridge Univ. Press.
Proust, M. 1981. *Remembrance of things past,* vol. I. New York: Random
House.
Raloff, J. 2000. Chocolate hearts: Yummy and good medicine? *Science
News* 157:188.
Raloff, J. 1999. Well-done research: New recipes for making seriously
browned meats less of a cancer risk. *Science News* 155:264.
Richer, C., Decker, N., Belin, J., Imbs, J. L., Montastruc, J. L., Giudicelli, J. F.
1989. Odorous urine in man after asparagus. *Br. J. Clin. Pharmacol.*
27:640.
Royal Institute of Chemistry. 1997. Garlic's healthy effects explained.
Chem. Br. 33(11):11.
Royal Institute of Chemistry. 1987. Microwaved bacon. *Chem. Br.* 23:1158.
Snyder, C. H. 1998. *The extraordinary chemistry of ordinary things.* New
York: John Wiley.
Waring, R. H., Mitchel, S. C., Fenwick, G. R. 1987. The chemical nature of
the urinary odor produced by man after asparagus ingestion. *Xenobiot-
ica* 17:1363.
Wu, C. 2000. Toxin in absinthe makes neurons run wild. *Science News*
157:214.

Chapter 2
Agosta, W. 1996. *Bombardier beetles and fever trees: A close-up look at
chemical warfare and signals in animals and plants.* Menlo Park,
Calif.: Addison-Wesley.
British Medical Association. 1997. *The therapeutic uses of cannabis.* Am-
sterdam: Harwood.
Clayman, C. B., ed. 1989. *Encyclopedia of medicine.* The American
Medical Association, New York: Random House, p. 583. Table of
viruses.
Cowley, G. The heart. *Newsweek,* Aug. 11, 1997, p. 52.
Emsley, J. 1998. *Molecules at an exhibition: The science of everyday life.*
Oxford: Oxford Univ. Press.
Emsley, J. 1994. *The consumer's good chemical guide: A jargon-free guide
to the chemicals of everyday life.* Oxford: W. H. Freeman.

Further Reading

Giovanni, A., Szallasi, A. 1997. Euphorbium: Modern research on its active principle, resineferatoxin, revives an ancient medicine. *Life Sci.* 60(10):681.

Goldstein, D. B. 1983. *Pharmacology of alcohol.* New York: Oxford Univ. Press.

Grady, D. Scientists say herbs need more regulation. *The New York Times,* Mar 7, 2000, p. 1 (Science section.)

Holland, B. K. 1996. *Prospecting for drugs in ancient and mediaeval European texts: A scientific approach.* Amsterdam: Harwood.

Judge, M. 1996. No pain, more gain. *New Scientist* 152(2058):30. (A review of antiinflammatory drugs.)

Levy, S. B. 1999. The challenge of antibiotic resistance. *Sci. Am.* 278(3):30.

Liska, K. 1990. *Drugs and the human body.* New York: Macmillan.

Mann, J., Crabbe, J. C. 1996. *Bacteria and antibacterial agents.* Oxford: Oxford Univ. Press.

Mann, J. 1994. *Murder, magic and medicine.* Oxford: Oxford Univ. Press.

New Scientist. 1998. Drug resistance in hospitals has been traced to the farmyard. *New Scientist* 157(2126):13. Editorial.

Ottoboni, M. A. 1991. *The dose makes the poison.* New York: Van Nostrand Reinhold.

Porter, R., Teich, M., eds. 1996. *Drugs and narcotics in history.* Cambridge: Cambridge Univ. Press.

Service, R. F. 1996. Closing in on a stomach-sparing aspirin substitute. *Science* 273:1660.

Snyder, C. H. 1998. *The extraordinary chemistry of ordinary things.* New York: John Wiley.

Stone, T., Darlington, G. 2000. *Pills potions poisons: How drugs work.* Oxford: Oxford Univ. Press.

Wainwright, M. 1990. *Miracle cure: The story of penicillin and the golden age of antibiotics.* Oxford: Blackwell.

Wilson, E. K. 1998. Impotence drugs: More than viagra. *Chem. Eng. News* 76(26):29.

Chapter 3

Culotta, E., Koshland, D. E. Jr. 1992. No news is good news. *Science* 258:1862.

Emsley, J. 1998. *Molecules at an exhibition: The science of everyday life.* Oxford: Oxford Univ. Press.

Emsley, J. 1994. *The consumer's good chemical guide: A jargon-free guide to the chemicals of everyday life.* Oxford: W. H. Freeman.

Fackelmann, K. 1997. Power failure: What happens when muscle cells run out of fuel. *Science News* 152:206.

Good, P. R., Geary, N., Engen, T. 1976. The effect of oestrogen on odour detection. *Chem. Senses Flavour* 2:45.

Grady, D. Scientists say herbs need more regulation. *The New York Times,* Mar 7, 2000, p. 1 (Science section.)

Graham, C. A., McGrew, W. C. 1980. Menstrual synchrony in female undergraduates living on a coeducational campus. *Psychoneuroendocrinology* 5:245.

Harvard Medical School. 2000. Supplements: A scorecard. *Harvard Men's Health Watch* 4(7):1.

Harvard Medical School. 1998. Vitamin D deficiency may be widespread. *Harvard Health Letter* 23(9):7.

Lagnado, L. Laetril makes a comeback on the web. *The Wall Street Journal,* Mar 22, 2000, p. B1.

Moore, P. 1996. Fueled for life, *Inside Science* 87:1; in *New Scientist* 149(2012). (Energy flow through plants and animals.)

Science Service. 1999. Some herbals may threaten fertility. *Science News* 155:207. (Report of mutation by St. John's Wort.)

Snyder, C. H. 1998. *The extraordinary chemistry of ordinary things.* New York: John Wiley.

Stone, T., Darlington, G. 2000. *Pills potions poisons: How drugs work.* Oxford: Oxford Univ. Press.

University of California. 1999. B_{12}: Don't B Deficient. *U. C. Berkeley Wellness Letter* 15(6):2.

Chapter 4

Baldry, P. E. 1976. *The battle against bacteria—A fresh look.* Cambridge: Cambridge Univ. Press.

Benjamin, D. R. 1995. *Mushrooms: Poisons and panaceas.* London: Freeman.

Brody, J. E. 1998. *Book of health.* New York: Times Books, Random House.

Cartwright, F. F. 1972. *Disease and history.* New York: Thomas Y. Crowell.

Clayman, C. B., ed. 1989. *Encyclopedia of medicine.* The American Medical Association, New York: Random House.

Cowley, G. The heart. *Newsweek,* Aug 11, 1997, p. 52.

Diamond, F. 1999. *Guns, germs, and steel: The fates of human societies.* New York: W. W. Norton.

Dixon, B. 1994. *Power unseen: How microbes rule the world.* Oxford: W. H. Freeman.

Dormandy, T. 1999. *The white death: A history of tuberculosis.* London: Hambledon Press.

Eley, A. R. 1996. *Microbial food poisoning.* London: Chapman & Hall.

Harris, J. B. 1986. *Natural toxins: Animal, plant, and microbial.* Oxford: Clarendon Press.

Levy, S. B. 1999. The challenge of antibiotic resistance. *Sci. Am.* 278(3):30.

Mann, J., Crabbe, J. C. 1996. *Bacteria and antibacterial agents.* Oxford: Oxford Univ. Press.

Mlot, C. 1997. The rise in toxic tides: What is behind the ocean blooms? *Science News* 152:202.

New Scientist. 1998. Drug resistance in hospitals has been traced to the farmyard. *New Scientist* 157(2126):13. Editorial.

Postgate, J. 1992. *Microbes and man.* London: Penguin Books.

Wainwright, M. 1990. *Miracle cure: The story of penicillin and the golden age of antibiotics.* Oxford: Blackwell.

Chapter 5

Abelson, P. H. 1995. Flaws in risk assessments. *Science* 270:215.

Abelson, P. H. 1994. Risk assessments of low-level exposures. *Science* 265:1507.

Ames, B. 1978. *Environmental chemicals causing cancer and genetic birth defects: Developing a strategy to minimize human exposure.* Berkeley: Institute of Governmental Studies, University of California.

Becker, Q. H. 1986. George Washington and variolation; Edward Jenner and vaccination. *J. Am. Med. Assoc.* 255(14):1881.

Brody, J. E., 1998. *Book of health.* New York: Times Books, Random House.

Brody, J. E., 1998. *Jane Brody's allergy fighter.* New York: W. W. Norton.

Cartwright, F. F. 1972. *Disease and history.* New York: Thomas Y. Crowell.

Clayman, C. B., ed. 1989. *Encyclopedia of medicine.* The American Medical Association, New York: Random House.

Culotta, E., Koshland, D. E. Jr. 1992. No news is good news. *Science* 258:1862.

Diamond, F. 1999. *Guns, germs, and steel: The fates of human societies.* New York: W. W. Norton.

Dormandy, T. 1999. *The white death: A history of tuberculosis.* London: Hambledon Press.

Emsley, J. 1994. *The consumer's good chemical guide: A jargon-free guide to the chemicals of everyday life.* Oxford: W. H. Freeman.

Estabrook, R. W. 1996. *Carcinogens and anticarcinogens in the human diet: A comparison of naturally occurring and synthetic substances.* Washington, DC: National Academy Press.

Evans, D. 1998. Agrochemicals: Benefits and risks. *Chem. Br.* 34(7):20.

Gray, H. B., Simon, J. D., Trogler, W. C. 1995. *Braving the elements.* Sausalito, Calif.: University Science Books.

Gribble, G. W. 1998. Dioxin discoveries. *Chem. Eng. News* 76(24):4.

Hileman, B., Long, J., Kirschner, E. M. 1994. Chlorine industry running flat out despite persistent health fears. *Chem. Eng. News* 72(47):12–22.

Hoekstra, E. J., de Leer, E. 1995. Organohalogens: The natural alternative. *Chem. Br.* 31:127.

Hogue, C. 2000. Identifying carcinogens. *Chem. Eng. News* 78(12):8.

Judge, M. 1996. No pain, more gain. *New Scientist* 152(2058):30. (A review of antiinflammatory drugs.)

Further Reading

Lederberg, J. 2000. Infectious history. *Science* 288:287.

Liska, K. 1990. *Drugs and the human body.* New York: Macmillan.

Oda, Y. 1999. Inoculation in Boston from 1721 to American independence. *Nippon Ishigaku Zasshi* 45(1):31–44 (In Japanese, English abstract).

Raloff, J. 1999. Redefining dioxins. *Science News* 155:156.

Raloff, J. 1999. Well-done research: New recipes for making seriously browned meats less of a cancer risk. *Science News* 155:264.

Rodricks, J. V. 1992. *Calculated risks: Understanding the toxicity and health risks of chemicals in our environment.* Cambridge: Cambridge Univ. Press.

Salzberg, H. W. 1991. *From caveman to chemist: Circumstances and achievements.* Washington, DC: American Chemistry Society.

Snyder, C. H. 1998. *The extraordinary chemistry of ordinary things.* New York: John Wiley.

Stone, R. 1995. A molecular approach to cancer risk. *Science* 268:356.

Stone, T., Darlington, G. 2000. *Pills potions poisons: How drugs work.* Oxford: Oxford Univ. Press.

Trefil, J. 1996. *101 things you don't know about science and no one else does either.* New York: Houghton Mifflin.

University of California. 2000. Does this mineral (selenium) prevent cancer? *U. C. Berkeley Wellness Letter* 16(9):1.

University of California. 2000. Living by the numbers: How to gauge your risks. *U. C. Berkeley Wellness Letter* 16(9):4.

Weinberg, R. A. 1998. *One renegade cell: How cancer begins.* New York: Basic Books.

Chapter 6

Abelson, P. H. 1994. Chlorine and organochlorine compounds. *Science* 265:1153.

Bast, J. L., Hill, P. J., Rue, R. C. 1994. *Eco-sanity: A common-sense guide to environmentalism.* Lanham, MD: Madison Books.

da Silva, J. J. R. F., Williams, R. J. P. 1991. *The biological chemistry of the elements.* Oxford: Clarendon Press.

Emsley, J. 1998. *Molecules at an exhibition: The science of everyday life.* Oxford: Oxford Univ. Press.

Emsley, J. 1994. *The consumer's good chemical guide: A jargon-free guide to the chemicals of everyday life.* Oxford: W. H. Freeman.

Gray, H. B., Simon, J. D., Trogler, W. C. 1995. *Braving the elements.* Sausalito, Calif.: University Science Books.

Greenwood, N. N., Earnshaw, A. 1984. *Chemistry of the elements.* Oxford: Pergamon Press.

Gribble, G. W. 1998. Dioxin discoveries. *Chem. Eng. News* 76(24):4.

Hamilton G. 1998. Open wide, we are going to explore. *New Scientist* 157(2125):32. (Fighting Tooth Decay.)

Hileman, B. 2000. Tetraethyllead versus ethanol: A precautionary tale. *Chem. Eng. News* 78(16):29.

Hileman, B., Long, J., Kirschner, E. M. 1994. Chlorine industry running flat out despite persistent health fears. *Chem. Eng. News* 72(47):12–22.

Hoekstra, E. J., de Leer, E. 1995. Organohalogens: The natural alternative. *Chem. Br.* 31:127.

Hughes, J. T. 1992. *Aluminium and your health*. Cirencester, UK: Rimes House.

Kollerstrom, N. 1982. *Lead on the brain*. London: Wildwood House.

Kutsky, R. J. 1981. *Handbook of vitamins, minerals and hormones*. New York: Van Nostrand Reinhold.

MacKenzie, D. 1995. Cleaning crops with cleanliness. *New Scientist* 147(1996):4.

Monastersky, R. 1998. The ice that burns. *Science News* 154:312. (Methane hydrates.)

Pearce, F. 1997. Planet Earth is drowning in nitrogen. *New Scientist* 154(2077):10.

Pearce, F. 1996. Finnish study challenges radon's deadly reputation. *New Scientist* 151(2040):8.

Raloff, J. 1999. Well-done research: New recipes for making seriously browned meats less of a cancer risk. *Science News* 155:264.

Salzberg, H. W. 1991. *From caveman to chemist: Circumstances and achievements*. Washington, DC: American Chemistry Society.

Senozan, N. M., Devore, J. A. 1996. Carbon monoxide poisoning. *J. Chem. Edu.* 73(3):767.

Silvester, M. J. 1993. Landmarks in organofluorine chemistry. *Chem. Br.* 29:215–218.

Snyder, C. H. 1998. *The extraordinary chemistry of ordinary things*. New York: John Wiley.

Thompson, K. 1989. Copper in the diet. *Chem. Br.* 25:855.

University of California. 2000. Does this mineral (selenium) prevent cancer? *U. C. Berkeley Wellness Letter* 16(9):1.

University of California. 1999. B_{12}: Don't B deficient. *U. C. Berkeley Wellness Letter* 15(6):2.

Wells, W. 2000. From explosives to the gas that heals: Nitric oxide in biology and medicine. *Beyond Discovery*, Washington, DC: National Academy of Sciences. (www.beyonddiscovery.org)

Chapter 7

Abelson, P. H. 1994. Chlorine and organochlorine compounds. *Science* 265:1153.

Adams, M. G. 1980. Odour producing organs of mammals. *Symp. Zool. Soc. London.* 45:57.

Agosta, W. C. 1992. *Chemical communication: The language of pheromones*. New York: Scientific American Library.

Allardice, P. 1989. *Aphrodisiacs and love magic. The mystic lure of love charms*. Dorset, UK: Prism Press.

Ayabe-Kanamura, S., Schicker, I., Lasker, M., Hudson, R., Distel, H., Kobayakawa, T., Saito, S. 1998. Differences in perception of everyday odors: A Japanese–German cross-cultural study. *Chem. Senses* 23:31.

Bast, J. L., Hill, P. J., Rue, R. C. 1994. *Eco-sanity: A common-sense guide to environmentalism*. Lanham, MD: Madison Books.

Berliner, D. L., Monti-Bloch, L., Jennings-White, C., Diaz-Sanchez, V. 1996. The functionality of the human vomeronasal organ (VNO): Evidence for steroid receptors. *J. Steroid Biochem. Molec. Biol.* 58:26.

Bucherl, W., ed. 1968. *Venomous animals and their venoms*. New York: Academic Press.

Cernoch, J. M., Porter, R. H. 1985. Recognition of maternal axillary odors by infants. *Child Devel.* 56:1593.

Comfort, A. 1971. Likelihood of human pheromones. *Nature* 230:432.

Committee on Comparative Toxicity of Naturally Occurring Carcinogens, National Research Council. 1996. *Carcinogens and anticarcinogens in the human diet: A comparison of naturally occurring and synthetic substances*. Washington, DC: National Academy Press.

Doty, R. L. 1982. Communications of gender from human breath odors. *Horm. Behav.,* 16:13.

Edstrom, A. 1992. *Venomous and poisonous animals*. Malabar, Fla.: Krieger.

Eley, A. R. 1996. *Microbial food poisoning*. London: Chapman & Hall.

Emsley, J. 1998. *Molecules at an exhibition: The science of everyday life*. Oxford: Oxford Univ. Press.

Emsley, J. 1994. *The consumer's good chemical guide: A jargon-free guide to the chemicals of everyday life*. Oxford: W. H. Freeman.

Evans, D. 1998. Agrochemicals: Benefits and risks. *Chem. Br.* 34(7):20.

Giovanni, A., Szallaski, A. 1997. Euphorbium: Modern research on its active principle, resineferatoxin, revives an ancient medicine. *Life Sci.* 60(10):681.

Good, P. R., Geary, N., Engen, T. 1976. The effect of oestrogen on odour detection. *Chem. Senses Flav.* 2:45.

Graham, C. A., McGrew, W. C. 1980. Menstrual synchrony in female undergraduates living on a coeducational campus. *Psychoneuroendocrinology* 5:245.

Gray, H. B., Simon, J. D., Trogler, W. C. 1995. *Braving the elements*. Sausalito, Calif.: University Science Books.

Gribble, G. W. 1998. Dioxin discoveries. *Chem. Eng. News* 76(24):4.

Hanson, D. 1999. MTBE: Villain or victim? *Chem. Eng. News* 77(42):49.

Harris, J. B. 1986. *Natural toxins: Animal, plant, and microbial.* Oxford: Clarendon Press.

Harte, J. 1988. *Consider a spherical cow.* Sausalito, Calif.: University Science Books.

Hasler, A. D., Larson, J. A. 1958. The homing salmon. *Sci. Am.* 202:72.

Hileman, B. 2000. Tetraethyllead versus ethanol: A precautionary tale. *Chem. Eng. News* 78(16):29.

Hileman, B., Long, J., Kirschner, E. M. 1994. Chlorine industry running flat out despite persistent health fears. *Chem. Eng. News* 72(47):12–22.

Hoekstra, E. J., de Leer, E. 1995. Organohalogens: The natural alternative. *Chem. Br.* 31:127.

Kalmus, H. 1955. The discrimination by the nose of the dog of individual human odours and in particular the odour of twins. *Br. J. Anim. Behav.* 3:25.

Kotulak, R. 1996. *Inside the brain: Revolutionary discoveries of how the mind works.* Kansas City, Mo.: Andrews and McMeel.

MacKenzie, D. 1995. Cleaning crops with cleanliness. *New Scientist* 147(1996):4.

Mlot, C. 1997. The rise in toxic tides: What is behind the ocean blooms? *Science News* 152:202.

Pearce, F. 1997. Planet Earth is drowning in nitrogen. *New Scientist* 154(2077):10.

Pfeiffer, W. 1963. Alarm substances. *Experientia* 19:113.

Proust, M. 1981. *Remembrance of things past,* vol. I. New York: Random House.

Raloff, J. 1999. Redefining dioxins. *Science News* 155:156.

Smith, K., Sines, J. O. 1960. Demonstration of a peculiar odor in the sweat of schizophrenic patients. *Arch. Gen. Psych.* 2:184.

Snyder, C. H. 1998. *The extraordinary chemistry of ordinary things.* New York: John Wiley.

Stern, K., McClintock, M. K. 1998. Regulation of ovulation by human pheromones. *Nature* 292:177.

Stoddart, D. M. 1990. *The scented ape: The biology and culture of human odour.* Cambridge: Cambridge Univ. Press.

Taberner, P. V. 1985. *Aphrodisiacs: The science and the myth.* London: Croom Helm.

Taylor, R. 1997. The sixth sense. *New Scientist* 153(2066):36. (Discussion of the vomeronasal organ and human behavior.)

Watson, L. 2000. *Jacobson's organ and the remarkable nature of smell.* New York: W. W. Norton.

Weller, A. 1999. Communication through body odour. *Nature* 392:126.

Wells, W. 2000. From explosives to the gas that heals: Nitric oxide in biology and medicine. *Beyond Discovery,* Washington, DC: National Academy of Sciences. (www.beyonddiscovery.org)

Chapter 8

Balling, R. C. 1992. *The heated debate: Greenhouse predictions versus climate reality.* San Francisco: Pacific Research Institute for Public Policy. (The author believes we are far from environmental disaster.)

Bast, J. L., Hill, P. J., Rue, R. C. 1994. *Eco-sanity: A common-sense guide to environmentalism.* Lanham, MD: Madison Books.

Calvin. W. H. The great climate flip-flop. *The Atlantic Monthly,* Jan 1998, p. 47.

Gelbspan, R. 1997. *The heat is on: The high stakes battle over Earth's threatened climate.* Reading, Mass.: Addison-Wesley. (The author argues the energy industry has created an appearance of uncertainty about global warming in order to slow policy response to the changes.)

Gray, H. B., Simon, J. D., Trogler, W. C. 1995. *Braving the elements.* Sausalito, Calif.: University Science Books.

Hansen, J. E., Sato, M., Reudy, R., Lacis, A., Glascoe, J. 1998. Global climate data and models: A reconciliation. *Science* 281:930.

Harte, J. 1988. *Consider a spherical cow.* Sausalito, Calif.: University Science Books.

Hileman, B. 1997. Industry considers CO_2 reduction methods. *Chem. Eng. News* 75(26):30.

McGuire, B. 1997. Blowing hot and cold. *New Scientist* 156(2103):32. (Volcanoes and global warming.)

McKibben, B. 1989. *The end of nature.* New York: Random House. (The author describes the seriousness of global climate change and the need to adjust how we live to prevent destruction of our world.)

Michaels, P. J. 1992. *Sound and fury: The science and politics of global warming.* Washington, DC: Cato Institute. (The author is an outspoken "greenhouse skeptic" arguing that global warming is a political, not scientific, issue.)

Monastersky, R. 1998. The ice that burns. *Science News* 154:312. (Methane hydrates.)

Pearce, F. 1997. Planet Earth is drowning in nitrogen. *New Scientist* 154(2077):10.

Pearce, F. 1997. Aircraft wreak havoc on ozone layer. *New Scientist* 153(2069):18.

Schneider, S. H. 1997. *Laboratory Earth: The planetary gamble we can't afford to lose.* New York: Harper Collins. (The author argues that the United States is slow to respond to anthropological changes in the Earth's climate.)

Singer, F. S. 1997. *Hot air, cold science: Global warming's unfinished debate.* Oakland, Calif.: Independent Institute. (The author describes the lack of consensus even among scientists on many issues of global warming.)

Further Reading

Snyder, C. H. 1998. *The extraordinary chemistry of ordinary things.* New York: John Wiley.

Trefil, J. 1996. *101 things you don't know about science and no one else does either.* New York: Houghton Mifflin.

Chapter 9

Bower, B. 1998. Bright lights dim winter depression. *Science News* 154: 260.

Gray, H. B., Simon, J. D., Trogler, W. C. 1995. *Braving the elements.* Sausalito, Calif.: University Science Books.

Raloff, J. 2000. Two studies offer some cell-phone cautions. *Science News* 157:328.

Raloff, J. 1998. Does light have a dark side? Nighttime illumination might elevate cancer risk. *Science News* 154:248.

Raloff, J. 1998. EMFs' biological influences. *Science News* 153:29.

Chapter 10

Abelson, P. H. 1996. Nuclear power in East Asia. *Science* 272:465.

Gray, H. B., Simon, J. D., Trogler, W. C. 1995. *Braving the elements.* Sausalito, Calif.: University Science Books.

Hart, M. M. 1997. Radiation—What is important? *Radiation Safety Officer,* March/April, p. 27.

Hileman, B. 1994. US and Russia face urgent decisions on weapons plutonium. *Chem. Eng. News* 77(24):12–25.

Pearce, F. 1996. Finnish study challenges radon's deadly reputation. *New Scientist* 151(2040):8.

Rhodes, R. 1986. *The making of the atomic bomb.* New York: Simon & Schuster.

Glossary

A

absorption Any process by which a substance incorporates another into itself, or takes in radiant or sound energy.

acetaldehyde CH_3CHO, industrial chemical, product of ethanol metabolism in humans.

acetic acid CH_3COOH, known as vinegar in the dilute form; a common intermediate in cellular metabolism.

acid A substance that increases the hydrogen ion concentration when dissolved in water.

acid rain Precipitation that is acidic; the acidity results from reactions between water droplets and atmospheric sulfur dioxide (producing sulfuric acid) and nitrogen dioxide (producing nitric acid).

active site The portion of an enzyme that attaches to the substrate by means of weak chemical bonds.

adenine A nitrogenous base found in DNA and RNA. In DNA, it pairs with thymine. In RNA, it pairs with uracil.

aerobic *(air-OH-bik)* An organism, environment, or cellular process that requires oxygen.

aflatoxin B_1 A toxic molecule and suspected carcinogen produced by molds in many foods.

AIDS (acquired immunodeficiency syndrome) The later stages of HIV infection; defined by a specified reduction of T cells and the appearance of characteristic secondary infections.

alcohol dehydrogenase An enzyme that breaks down alcohols.

alcohol group A hydroxyl group (OH) bound to a carbon atom.

alcohols A class of compounds of general formula ROH, with a hydroxyl group (OH) bonded to a carbon atom.

aldehydes A class of highly reactive organic compounds of general formula RCHO, containing a carbonyl group.

alkali A water-soluble compound of an alkali metal (e.g., Li, Na, K, Rb, Cs) or ammonia. Alkalis neutralize acids to form salts and turn red litmus paper blue.

alkaline solution A solution containing a basic substance.

alkaloid A nitrogen-containing organic compound found in plants that is basic, tastes bitter, and is often poisonous (examples include cocaine and quinine).

allele *(uh-LEEL)* An alternative form of a gene.

allergy A hypersensitivity to a specific substance (e.g., a food, pollen, dust) that is an overreaction by the body's immune response.

allotrope One of the two or more forms of an element; allotropes differ in their crystalline or molecular structure.

alloy A substance composed of two or more metals.

alpha-helix A coiled, rodlike structure formed by segments of an amino acid chain in the folded three-dimensional structure of a protein.

alpha-particle Helium nuclei emitted from radioactive materials undergoing alpha disintegration.

aluminum Al, element 13 of the periodic table; a common structural metal.

Ames test A bacterial bioassay for detecting mutagenic compounds; developed by Bruce Ames in 1974.

amide bond (link) A chemical bond formed between a carboxylic group (CO_2H) and an amine group (NH_2). Amide bonds connect individual amino acids into peptides and proteins.

amides A class of compounds derived from carboxylic acids and ammonia.

amino acid A general class of organic molecules containing a NH_2 group and a COOH group; the 20 different amino acids are the building blocks of proteins.

ammonia NH_3; a basic chemical and the main nitrogen source for fertilizers.

ammonium NH_4^+, protonated form of ammonia.

anabolic steroid A synthetic hormone that aids in tissue building.

anaerobic *(an-air-OH-bik)* Referring to an organism, environment, or cellular process that lives without oxygen and may be poisoned by it.

analytic chemistry Study of the compounds or elements comprising a chemical substance.

anemia A condition in which the blood is deficient in red blood cells, in hemoglobin, or in volume.

anion A negatively charged atom or molecule.

antibiotic A chemical that kills or inhibits the growth of bacteria.

antibody A protein formed by an animal in response to invasion by a foreign substance or cell (an antigen) that binds with that substance or cell and neutralizes or kills it.

antioxidant A molecule that blocks oxidation (an example is vitamin E).

arginine One of the 20 amino acids in proteins.

aromatic hydrocarbons A special class of cyclic polyunsaturated compounds; a typical example is benzene.

arsenic   As, element 33 of the periodic table; a poisonous heavy metal.

artery   A vessel that carries blood away from the heart.

arthritis, rheumatoid   An inflammatory joint disease thought to involve an autoimmune reaction.

aspartic acid   One of the 20 amino acids used in proteins.

aspirin   Acetylsalicylic acid; analgesic made from phenol.

atom   The fundamental building block of an element.

atomic number   The number of protons in the nucleus of an atom; unique for each element and designated by a subscript to the left of the elemental symbol.

ATP (adenosine triphosphate) *(uh-DEN-ohsin try-FOS-fate)*   An organic compound that releases energy when its last two phosphate bonds are hydrolyzed; this energy is used to drive reactions in cells.

autoimmune disease   Any of a group of diseases (e.g., juvenile diabetes, lupus, rheumatoid arthritis) that involve the formation of antibodies against antigens produced by the person's own body.

azides   Salts of an acid, HN_3, usually shock-explosive (*see* sodium azide).

B

bacterium (plural, **bacteria**)   A single-celled microorganism, also called a prokaryote, that has no true nucleus; bacteria are classified into two groups based on a difference in cell walls.

baking powder   A mixture of baking soda and a weak acid that causes rapid release of carbon dioxide when dissolved in water.

baking soda $NaHCO_3$; sodium bicarbonate; a weak base used to neutralize stomach acid; releases carbon dioxide gas on protonation, which causes baked goods to rise.

base   A substance that increases the concentration of OH^- ions in water; accepts protons and neutralizes an acid. Bases generally have a bitter taste and are slippery to the touch.

battery   A device that converts chemical energy into electricity.

beta-carotene   An antioxidant and precursor to vitamin A; found in carrots.

beta-decay   Radioactive decay process in which the nucleus of an element ejects an electron.

beta-particle   An electron ejected from an atomic nucleus during ß-decay.

beta-ray   A stream of electrons or positrons emitted from radioactive nuclei.

biochemicals   Molecules that participate in the chemical reactions of living systems.

biochemistry   The study of the chemical processes of living systems.

biological species   A group whose members can interbreed.

bioluminescence   Biochemical reaction in which chemical energy is converted into light; for example, the light of a firefly.

bleach   Chemical that oxidizes and removes colored impurities;

combustion The heat-releasing reaction between oxygen in air and a substance; burning.

concentration A measure of the number of molecules of a substance dissolved in a fixed volume of solvent.

condensation The change of a substance from a gaseous to a liquid or solid state.

crystal A solid formed by the regular stacking of atoms or molecules in a three-dimensional solid.

cubic centimeter Volume of a cube with edges 1 centimeter long; equals 1 milliliter.

cyanide CN^-; a weak base that is highly toxic.

cytochrome *c* oxidase An important enzyme of the respiratory cycle of some aerobic organisms (including humans) that catalyzes the reduction of oxygen to water.

D

DDT A pesticide banned in the United States but still used in many countries throughout the world. While it was in use, the worldwide incidence of malaria decreased greatly, but since its ban, the incidence has been on the increase.

dental amalgam Alloy of silver, mercury, copper, and tin used to fill cavities in teeth.

deoxyribose The sugar component of DNA; has one less hydroxyl group than ribose, the sugar component of RNA.

deuterium ^2H or D; the hydrogen isotope in which the nucleus contains one proton and one neutron.

diethylene glycol $HOCH_2CH_2OCH_2CH_2OH$; a toxic industrial solvent.

dipole (electric) The net separation of positive and negative charge in a molecule.

disaccharide *(dy-SAK-ur-ide)* A double sugar, consisting of two monosaccharides.

distillation A process used to separate the components of a liquid mixture; the liquid is heated and escaping vapors collected and recondensed and collected by cooling the vapors over a different container.

DNA Deoxyribonucleic acid; the molecule that stores all genetic information in cells. *See* recombinant DNA.

double bond A strong bond between two atoms that consists of four shared electrons.

E

electric charge An inherent property of matter; electrons carry a negative charge and nuclei normally carry a similar positive charge for each electron in the atom.

electromagnetic spectrum All wavelengths of electromagnetic radiation, including radio waves, microwaves, infrared light, visible light, ultraviolet light, X-rays, and gamma rays.

electron   A negatively charged particle of low mass that makes up part of an atom.

element   Simple substance composed of atoms of the same atomic number.

endorphin *(en-DOR-fin)*   A hormone produced in the brain and anterior pituitary that inhibits pain perception.

energy   The capacity to do work by moving matter against an opposing force.

enzyme   A protein that catalyzes a chemical reaction.

esters   Organic compounds formed by condensation of an acid with an alcohol with the elimination of water.

estrogens *(ES-troh-jens)*   The primary female steroid sex hormones, they stimulate the development and maintenance of the female reproductive system and secondary sex characteristics.

ethanol CH_3CH_2OH; a gasoline additive and an intoxicating component in alcoholic beverages.

ethers   A class of organic compounds containing an oxygen atom attached to two carbon atoms.

ethyl compounds   Organic compounds containing the ethyl group C_2H_5.

ethylene glycol   A viscous, toxic alcohol used as a component in antifreeze and sometimes illegally added to wine to enhance its sweetness.

eukaryotic cell *(YOO-kar-ee-OT-ik)*   A cell with a membrane-enclosed nucleus and membrane-enclosed organelles; present in protists, plants, fungi, and animals.

evaporation   The process by which molecules on the surface of a liquid absorb heat and enter the gas phase.

evaporative cooling   The property of a liquid whereby the surface becomes cooler during evaporation, owing to a loss of highly energetic molecules to the gaseous state.

F

Fahrenheit   A temperature scale used in the English system. Water freezes at 32 °F and boils at 212 °F.

fat (triacylglycerol) *(tri-AH-sil-GLIS-er-all)*   A biological compound consisting of three fatty acids linked to one glycerol molecule.

fats   Naturally occurring organic molecules that consist primarily of hydrocarbon chains. Common fats are butter, lard, margarine, olive oil, corn oil, and beef tallow.

fatty acid   A long-carbon-chain carboxylic acid. Fatty acids vary in length and in the number and location of double bonds; three fatty acids linked to a glycerol molecule form fat.

FDA: The US Food and Drug Administration, the federal agency that sets standards for, and approves claims about, the efficacy and safety of drugs and the quality of foods.

fentanyl   A potent narcotic used to relieve postsurgical pain.

fermentation   A catabolic process that makes a limited amount of ATP from glucose and that produces a characteristic end product, such as ethyl alcohol or lactic acid.

fertilizer   Chemical applied to soil that provides the nitrogen, phosphorus, and potassium atoms that are essential for plant growth.

fluorine   F; element 9 of the periodic table. Fluorine gas (F_2) is a powerful oxidant.

folic acid   One of the B vitamins; widely distributed in vegetable and animal foods, and active as a coenzyme in many metabolic pathways in all cells.

force   In mechanics, the physical quantity that, when it acts on a body, causes it to change its state of motion or tends to deform it.

formaldehyde   The very simple organic molecule H_2CO, commonly used to disinfect and to preserve biological specimens. It is also an active intermediate in cellular metabolism.

free radical   A molecule or atom that has one unpaired electron.

freezing point   The temperature at which a liquid solidifies.

Freon   One of a class of fluorocarbons or chlorofluorocarbons.

frequency   The rate at which a wave motion completes its cycle; measured in hertz (Hz).

fructose   A sugar found in fruits.

G

gamma rays   High-energy photons emitted from atomic nuclei during radioactive decay.

gas   One of the three states of matter; a low-density material that expands to fill its container.

gasoline   A mixture of hydrocarbons derived from oil that boils between 40 °C and 180 °C.

gene   A sequence of DNA that encodes the information for a protein or an RNA; a unit of heredity at a specific place on a chromosome.

genome *(JEE-nome)*   The complete complement of an organism's genes.

gland   An organ that extracts specific substances from the blood and concentrates or alters them for future secretion.

glass   A rigid material that has no well-defined structure. Common glass consists of silica (SiO_2), limestone ($CaCO_3$), and sodium carbonate (Na_2CO_3).

global warming   The increase in the Earth's average temperature as a result of increases in the concentrations of greenhouse gases.

glucose   A 6-carbon sugar that provides the main fuel for cellular respiration.

glutamic acid   One of the 20 amino acids used in proteins.

Glossary

glycine   The simplest of the 20 amino acids in proteins.

glycogen *(GLY-koh-jen)*   An extensively branched, glucose-storage polysaccharide found in the liver and muscle of animals; the animal equivalent of starch.

gram   A measure of weight equivalent to 0.0352 ounce.

graphite   A solid form of carbon in which the carbon atoms are linked in hexagonal planar arrays. Because these layered sheets are not covalently bonded to one another, this material is a good lubricant and constitutes the "lead" in pencils.

greenhouse effect   The warming of planet Earth as the result of the atmospheric accumulation of carbon dioxide and other gases that absorb infrared radiation and slow its escape from the Earth.

greenhouse gases   Chemicals in the atmosphere that absorb the infrared radiation (heat) emitted by the Earth. These include carbon dioxide, water, nitrous oxide, chlorofluorocarbons, and methane.

H

half-life   The time required for a reaction to proceed halfway to completion, commonly used as a measure of radioactive decay times.

halogens   Elements in column 17 of the periodic table that includes fluorine (F), chlorine (Cl), bromine (Br), iodine (I), and astatine (At).

heat   A form of energy that passes from one body to another because of a temperature difference between them.

heat of combustion   The heat released when a substance is burned in oxygen.

helium   He; element 2 of the periodic table; an inert gas that is lighter than air; produced in the Earth by α-decay.

hemoglobin *(HEE-moh-gloh-bin)*   An iron-containing protein in red blood cells that reversibly binds oxygen.

herbicide   A chemical that interferes with the growth of plants; used to control weeds.

heroin   An addictive narcotic made by adding a group from acetic acid to morphine.

heterogeneous   Referring to a system in which more than one phase is involved.

heterogeneous catalysis   A reaction wherein the catalyst is in a different phase from the reactants or products.

heterozygous *(HET-ur-oh-ZY-gus)*   Having two different alleles for a given trait.

homeostasis *(HOME-ee-oh-STAY-sis)*   The relatively constant physiological state of the body.

homocysteine   An amino acid for which the level in the blood is thought to correlate with heart problems.

hormones   Compounds that carry regulatory signals from one cell or tissue to another.

Glossary

Human Genome Project   An international collaborative effort to map and sequence the DNA of the human genome.

hydrocarbon *(HY-droh-kar-bon)*   An organic molecule consisting only of carbon and hydrogen.

hydrochloric acid   HCl; a strong industrial acid; the acid of the stomach.

hydrofluoric acid   HF; a highly toxic acid used in oil refining and in etching glass and silicon.

hydrogen   H; element 1 of the periodic table; exists naturally as H_2, a highly flammable gas.

hydrogen cyanide   HCN; a deadly gas.

hydrogen ion   A single proton with a charge of +1. The dissociation of a water molecule (H_2O) generates one hydroxide ion (OH^-) and a hydrogen ion (H^+).

hydrogen peroxide H_2O_2; a strong oxidant and bleaching agent available in drugstores as a weak 3% solution in water.

hydrogenation   Addition of hydrogen to carbon–carbon double or triple bonds; this reaction converts unsaturated fats and oils to saturated ones.

hydrophilic *(HY-droh-FIL-ik)*   Having an affinity for water.

hydrophobic *(HY-droh-FOH-bik)*   Having an aversion to water; tending to coalesce and form droplets in water.

hydroxide OH^-; a strong base.

hydroxyl group *(hy-DROKS-ul)*   An OH group bound to any other element through the oxygen atom.

I

inert   Unreactive.

infrared radiation   The part of the electromagnetic spectrum that extends from just below the visible to the microwave portions and thus has less energy than visible light but more energy than microwave. Although it is invisible to the eye, humans can detect infrared radiation by the sensation of warmth.

insulator   A substance that does not conduct electricity.

insulin   A hormone involved in glucose metabolism; a deficiency of insulin causes diabetes.

iodine   I; element 53 of the periodic table; an essential element in human nutrition.

ion   An atom or group of atoms that has become electrically charged by the gain or loss of electrons.

ionization   The dissociation of a neutral substance into positive and negative ions when the substance dissolves in water. For gases, the creation of a positive ion by loss of an electron.

iron   Fe; element 26 of the periodic table; an abundant metal essential for life.

isomer *(EYE-suh-mer)*   One of several organic compounds with the same molecular formula but different structures and therefore different properties. The three types of isomers are structural isomers, geometric isomers, and enantiomers.

isotope *(EYE-so-tope)*   One of several atomic forms of an element, each containing a different number of neutrons and thus differing in atomic mass (e.g., tritium and deuterium are isotopes of hydrogen).

J

joule (J)   A unit of energy; 1 J = 0.239 cal; 1 cal = 4.184 J.

K

kcal (kilocalorie)   One thousand calories; the amount of heat energy required to raise the temperature of 1 kg of water 1°C; equal to one nutritional Calorie.

kilometer   A measure of distance equal to 1,000 meters, or 0.62 mile.

L

laughing gas   *See* nitrous oxide.

lead   Pb; element 82 of the periodic table; the anode (reductant) in a car battery; a toxic heavy metal.

leaded gasoline   Gasoline that contains the octane enhancer tetraethyl lead.

lime   CaO; a weak base used in steel and cement manufacturing.

limestone $CaCO_3$; may also contain $MgCO_3$; when heated, it makes lime and releases carbon dioxide.

lipid *(LIH-pid)*   One of a family of compounds, including fats, phospho-lipids, and steroids, that are insoluble in water.

lipoprotein   A protein bonded to a lipid; includes the low-density lipoproteins (LDLs) and high-density lipoproteins (HDLs) that transport fats and cholesterol in blood.

liquid   One of the three states of matter. A liquid adopts the shape of the container but does not expand to fill it. Liquids are nearly as dense as solids, but they differ in that the molecules are not arranged in a regular fashion.

liter   A measure of liquid volume; equals 1,000 cubic centimeters or 1,000 milliliters; 1 liter equals 1.06 quarts.

lithium   Li; element 3 of the periodic table; lithium salts are used in the treatment of mental illness.

lysine   One of the 20 amino acids in proteins.

M

Manhattan Project   The top-secret US effort during World War II to build an atomic bomb.

mass   A measure of the amount of matter in a body.

matter Anything that takes up space and has mass.

mechanics Branch of applied mathematics dealing with the action of forces on bodies.

melanin The dark pigments in human skin; the tanning of skin involves the biosynthesis of melanin in response to exposure to ultraviolet rays in sunlight.

melting point The temperature at which a material changes from a solid to a liquid state.

metabolism *(meh-TAB-oh-liz-um)* All the chemical reactions of the body.

metal A solid characterized by its metallic luster, high thermal and electrical conductivities, and flexibility. Its unique properties result from the electrons being delocalized throughout the entire piece of metal.

methane CH_4; swamp gas; the simplest hydrocarbon and the primary component in natural gas.

methanol CH_3OH; wood alcohol; the simplest alcohol; a proposed alternative to gasoline; causes blindness, convulsion, and death when ingested as an impurity in moonshine.

methionine One of the 20 amino acids in proteins; it is one of two that contain sulfur.

methyl group The CH_3 group attached to an organic compound.

methyl-*t*-butyl ether MTBE; an octane enhancer in unleaded gasoline.

micro- A prefix meaning one-millionth.

microgram 0.000001 gram, or one-millionth of a gram.

micrometer 0.000001 meter, or one-millionth of a meter.

microwave radiation The part of the electromagnetic spectrum between infrared light and radio waves; used to heat food by exciting water molecules; used in telecommunications.

milli- A prefix meaning one-thousandth.

milligram (mg) 0.001 gram, or one-thousandth of a gram.

milliliter (ml) 0.001 liter, or one-thousandth of a liter; equals 1 cubic centimeter in volume.

millimeter (mm) 0.001 meter, or one-thousandth of a meter.

mirror image The reflected image of an object.

molecule Entity composed of atoms linked by chemical bonds and acting as a unit.

monosaccharide *(MON-oh-SAK-ur-ide)* The simplest carbohydrate; active alone or as a monomer for disaccharides and polysaccharides. Also known as simple sugars, the molecular formulas of monosaccharides are generally some multiple of CH_2O.

monounsaturated fat Fat in which the hydrocarbon chains contain one carbon−carbon double bond.

morphine An addictive narcotic pain reliever.

MTBE See Methyl-*t*-butyl ether.

mustard gas 2-chloroethyl sulfide; a chemotherapy agent and chemical weapon.

Glossary

mutagen *(MYOOT-uh-jen)* A chemical or physical agent that interacts with DNA and causes a mutation.

mutation *(myoo-TAY-shun)* A change in DNA caused by a mutagen.

myoglobin *(MY-uh-glow-bin)* An iron-containing protein that stores and releases oxygen in muscle tissues.

N

nano- Prefix meaning one-billionth.

natural gas Mixture of gaseous hydrocarbons found in underground deposits; consists primarily of methane.

nerve gas A substance that interferes with the transmission of nerve impulses; chemical warfare agent.

neurotransmitter A chemical that relays impulses between neurons or from neuron to muscle or gland.

neutralization A chemical reaction between compounds of opposite chemical character, giving an inactive product.

neutron A component of an atomic nucleus that has mass but no charge.

nicotine The addictive chemical in cigarettes; also a highly toxic chemical used as an insecticide.

nitrate NO_3^-; an anion with strong oxidizing properties.

nitrates Salts of nitric acid, containing the nitrate ion NO_3^-; almost all are soluble in water.

nitric acid HNO_3, a strong acid and strong oxidant used in the manufacture of fertilizers and explosives.

nitric oxide NO; a component in automobile exhaust, a neurotransmitter, and a deadly gas when inhaled.

nitrites Salts of nitrous acid, HNO_2.

nitrogen N; element 7 of the periodic table; naturally exists as the unreactive gas N_2; the primary constituent of the Earth's atmosphere.

nitrogen dioxide NO_2; the brown gaseous component of smog.

nitroglycerine A high explosive and heart medication.

nitrous oxide N_2O; a greenhouse gas and an anesthetic (laughing gas).

nonmetal A substance, particularly an element, showing none of the properties characteristic of metals.

nuclear waste Radioactive by-products from nuclear reactors.

nucleic acid RNA or DNA; polymers composed of monomers called nucleotides joined by covalent bonds between the phosphate of one nucleotide and the sugar of the next nucleotide.

nucleus (1) An atom's central core, containing protons and neutrons. (2) The membrane-bound chromosome-containing structure of a eukaryotic cell.

NutraSweet® The dipeptide Asp-Phe (aspartic acid-phenylalanine); a sugar substitute.

nylon A high-strength condensation polymer.

Glossary

O

oil   Any substance that is insoluble in water, soluble in ether, and greasy to the touch.

oncogene *(ON-koh-jeen)*   A gene that can trigger cancerous characteristics.

organic chemistry   The branch of chemistry pertaining to the study of carbon compounds containing hydrogen.

organic food   Food raised without use of synthetic fertilizers, herbicides, or pesticides.

organophosphates   A class of organic compounds containing phosphorus; used in pesticides (e.g., malathion).

osmotic pressure *(oz-MOT-ik)*   A measure of the tendency of a solution to take up water when separated from pure water by a selectively permeable membrane.

oxidant   Any compound that removes electrons from another compound (the reductant) in a chemical reaction.

oxidation   A chemical reaction in which electrons are removed from an atom or molecule; always accompanied by a reduction reaction.

oxide ion O^{2-}; a negatively charged ion present in many metal oxides.

oxidizing agent   Same as oxidant.

oxygen   O; element 8 of the periodic table; exists naturally as O_2 and O_3.

ozone O_3; a gas found in the stratosphere that protects the plants and animals on the surface of the Earth by filtering out the harmful ultraviolet light emitted by the sun; toxic to most forms of life. In the troposphere, ozone is formed in photochemical smog.

ozone hole   Area of ozone depletion in the stratosphere above Antarctica and the Arctic; caused by photochemical reactions of CFC molecules.

P

penicillin   An antibiotic that works by preventing the synthesis of bacterial cell walls.

peptide   A compound containing two or more amino acids.

periodic table   The chart that displays the elements in order of increasing atomic number; families of elements with similar properties are grouped in columns.

peroxide   Hydrogen peroxide, HOOH; a strong oxidizing and bleaching agent; refers to compounds containing an O-O bond.

pesticide   Chemical that kills pests (such as rats and insects).

PET   *See* positron emission tomography.

pH scale   A measure of hydrogen ion concentration equal to $-\log [H^+]$ and ranging in value from 0 to 14.

phenols   Class of aromatic compounds in which a hydroxide group is directly bonded to an aromatic ring system.

phenylalanine   One of the 20 amino acids in proteins.

pheromone *(FAIR-uh-mone)*   A small, volatile chemical that functions in communication between animals and acts much like a hormone in influencing physiology and behavior.

phosphates   Derivatives of phosphoric acid (H_3PO_4); either phosphate esters or salts containing phosphate ions (PO_4^{3-}).

phospholipids *(FOS-foh-LIP-ids)*   Molecules that constitute the inner bilayer of biological membranes; they have a polar, hydrophilic head and a nonpolar, hydrophobic tail.

photon *(FOH-tahn)*   The smallest particle that makes up light, whose energy content equals *hv*, where *h* is Planck's constant and *v* is the frequency of the light wave.

photosynthesis   The conversion of light energy to chemical energy stored in glucose or other organic compounds; occurs in plants, algae, and certain prokaryotes.

pineal gland *(PIN-ee-ul)*   Small endocrine gland in the vertebrate forebrain; secretes the hormone melatonin.

pituitary gland *(pih-TOO-ih-tair-ee)*   Endocrine gland at the base of the hypothalamus; consists of a posterior lobe (neurohypophysis), which stores and releases two hormones produced by the hypothalamus, and an anterior lobe (adenohypophysis), which produces and secretes many hormones that regulate diverse body functions.

plasminogen   Precursor of plasmin, an enzyme that dissolves blood clots.

plasminogen activator   A protease (protein-cleaving enzyme) that converts plasminogen to plasmin.

plastic   A solid, rigid polymer.

plasticizer   An organic compound added to a polymer to make it more flexible.

plutonium   Pu; element 94 in the periodic table; a synthetic element made by neutron bombardment of uranium. A fissionable radioactive substance used in breeder reactors and nuclear weapons.

poison ivy   The plant *Toxicodendron radicans;* oils from this plant contain urushiol, which causes an allergic reaction in the skin of many people.

polychlorinated biphenyls (PCBs)   A class of hazardous organic materials whose molecules contain two linked benzene rings with attached chlorine atoms; manufacture of PCBs has been banned in the United States since 1979, however, large amounts are still used today in a variety of industrial applications.

polysaccharide *(POL-ee-SAK-ur-ide)*   A polymer of many monosaccharides; formed by condensation synthesis.

porphyrin   An organic compound whose molecules contain four nitrogen atoms arranged in such a way that they can all simultaneously bind a metal ion (such as Fe^{2+}); this molecule occurs in heme proteins (such as myoglobin, hemoglobin, and cytochromes) and is responsible for their ability to transport and store O_2, as well as transfer electrons.

Glossary

positron   A positively charged electron; an example of antimatter. When a positron encounters a normal electron, they react immediately, and both particles are annihilated.

positron emission tomography (PET)   Medical imaging technique that measures gamma rays produced by positron-electron annihilation inside a patient's body to construct a three-dimensional image of organs.

potassium   K; element 19 of the periodic table; an element essential to life.

pressure   The force per unit area acting on a surface.

prion   An infectious form of protein that may increase in number by converting related proteins to more prions.

prokaryotic *(pro-KAR-ee-OT-ik)* **cell**   A type of cell lacking a membrane-enclosed nucleus and membrane-enclosed organelles; bacteria and archae are prokaryotic cells.

prostaglandin (PG) *(PROS-tuh-GLAN-din)*   One of a group of modified fatty acids secreted by virtually all tissues and performing a wide variety of functions as messengers.

proteins   Chains of 100 or more amino acids in a particular sequence that perform virtually all cellular functions, including those of enzymes, receptors, hormones, cytokines, interferons, and antibodies.

proton   A hydrogen ion, H^+; the positively charged component of an atomic nucleus.

R

radioactive dating   *See* carbon-14 dating.

radioactive isotope   An unstable isotope whose nucleus decays spontaneously, giving off detectable particles and energy.

radiocarbon dating   *See* carbon-14 dating.

radon   Rn; element 86 of the periodic table; a radioactive noble gas that is an environmental carcinogen.

reactant   A substance that undergoes a chemical reaction.

reagent   A substance that participates in a chemical reaction. Chemical reagents are commonly used to detect or determine another substance.

receptor   A molecule on the surface (membrane) of a cell that serves as a target for the binding of a hormone, drug, virus, or other entity that triggers a physiological or pharmacological response.

recombinant DNA   DNA created generally by genetic engineering, in which genetic sequences from diverse origins are joined together (recombined) to form a novel molecule.

reduction   A chemical process that adds electrons to an atom or molecule; often, one or more oxygen atoms are removed from the substance being reduced.

replication   The process by which a cell makes a copy of its DNA to pass on to its progeny.

retina *(REH-tin-uh)*   The innermost layer of the vertebrate eye, containing photoreceptor cells (rods and cones) and neurons; transmits images formed by the lens to the brain via the optic nerve.

retinol   Vitamin A.

retrovirus *(REH-troh-VY-rus)*   An RNA virus that reproduces by transcribing its RNA into DNA and then inserting the DNA into a cell; an important class of cancer-causing viruses.

ribose   The sugar component of nucleotides for RNA.

RNA: ribonucleic acid; a genetic molecule similar to DNA. RNA is constructed from a set of four building blocks called ribonucleotides, each consisting of a nitrogenous base (adenine, uracil, guanine, or cytosine), a sugar group (ribose), and a phosphate group. Many viruses use RNA instead of DNA to store genetic information.

rubber   An elastic polymer.

S

salicylates   Salts of salicylic acid, an aspirin derivative.

salt   A compound formed by neutralization of an acid and a base.

sand SiO_2; small grains of quartz.

sarin   A nerve gas.

saturated fat   A fat whose molecules contain only single bonds between adjacent carbon atoms.

sepsis   An acute and often fatal condition caused by infection, generally by gram-negative bacteria, leading to shock and multiple organ failure. No effective treatment is currently available.

silica   Silicon dioxide; SiO_2.

smog   A brown haze observed in industrialized areas that results from the presence and reactions of nitrogen dioxide in the atmosphere. Nitrogen dioxide is generated from oxidation of the nitric oxide emissions of automobiles. Photochemical reactions of nitrogen dioxide produce ozone.

soap   Alkali metal salts of fatty acids. These salts form micelles in water and act as cleaning agents.

sodium   Na; element 11 of the periodic table.

sodium azide   A salt, NaN_3, that forms nitrogen gas on heating; used to generate gas for rapid inflation of automotive airbags.

solar flare   Sudden, temporary outburst of energy from a small area on the sun's surface.

solar wind   Elementary particles (such as protons and electrons) that are continuously ejected from the Sun's surface into space.

solid   One of the three states of matter. A solid has a defined volume and space and is virtually incompressible; the atoms in a solid vibrate about fixed positions.

solubility   A measure of how much of a substance (the solute) can be dissolved in a solvent.

solution   A homogeneous molecular mixture of two or more substances, usually a solid and a liquid.

solvent   The liquid that dissolves a chemical substance; in a water solution of table salt, water is the solvent.

species   A particular kind of organism; members of the same species possess similar anatomical characteristics and have the ability to interbreed.

starch   A storage polysaccharide in plants consisting entirely of glucose.

steel   An alloy of iron, carbon, and other elements that is stronger and harder than pure iron.

steroid   A class of hormones whose molecules share a common structural backbone; most are derivatives of testosterone, the male sex hormone.

stratosphere   The region of the atmosphere that extends from the top of the troposphere to an altitude of about 50 km; this region contains the ozone layer.

sublimation   Transformation of a solid to the vapor state without an intervening liquid phase.

substrate   The substance on which an enzyme works.

sucrose   Common table sugar.

sugars   Sweet, soluble carbohydrates comprising the monosaccharides and the disaccharides.

sulfate SO_4^{2-}; an ion that occurs in many ionic solids and minerals.

sulfates   Salts of sulfuric acid; formed by reaction of the acid with metals, their oxides, or carbonates, or by oxidation of sulfides or sulfites.

sulfur   S; element 16 of the periodic table.

sulfur dioxide SO_2; a gas released in the burning of sulfur-containing coal and oil; reacts in the atmosphere to form acid rain.

sulfuric acid H_2SO_4; a strong acid and the largest volume industrial chemical in the world; chief component in acid rain.

sunscreens   Commercial chemical products that absorb ultraviolet light; the degree of protection depends on the concentration of the ultraviolet-absorbing molecule.

superoxide O_2^-; a destructive compound generated as a byproduct of aerobic metabolism.

T

Taxol   An anticancer drug that is isolated from the bark of the yew tree.

Teflon®   Addition polymer of tetrafluoroethylene, $F_2C=CF_2$, used as a nonstick coating and lubricant.

temperature   A measure of the intensity of heat in degrees; reflects the average kinetic energy of the molecules.

testosterone   The male sex hormone; a steroid; the most abundant androgen hormone in the male body.

Glossary

tetraethyllead $Pb(CH_2CH_3)_4$; an additive that increases the octane rating of gasoline.

tetrahydrocannabinol THC; the active ingredient in marijuana.

thalidomide A sedative that causes birth defects if taken by pregnant women.

thymus *(THY-mus)* An endocrine gland in the neck region of mammals that is active in establishing the immune system; secretes several messengers, including thymosin, that stimulate T cells.

thyroid gland An endocrine gland that secretes iodine-containing hormones (T_3 and T_4), which stimulate metabolism and influence development and maturation in vertebrates, and calcitonin, which lowers blood calcium levels in mammals.

tomography Imaging technique that creates a three-dimensional picture of an organ in the body.

tracer A radioactive element that is used in live subjects to study biological processes in the body, by, for example, positron emission tomography.

transferrin A protein that transports iron in the blood.

transformer A device for altering the voltage of an alternating current electricity supply.

transition elements (or transition metals) Elements (all metals) belonging to one of the following groups in the middle of the periodic table: 4, 5, 6, 7, 8, 9, 10, or 11.

triacylglycerol *(try-A-seel-gli-se-rol)* Chemical name for a fat molecule.

tritium ^3H, or T; the radioactive isotope of hydrogen; the ^3H nucleus contains one proton and two neutrons.

troposphere The layer of the atmosphere in contact with the Earth's surface; it extends 10 to 15 km above sea level.

tryptophan One of the 20 amino acids in proteins.

tumor A mass that forms within otherwise normal tissue caused by the uncontrolled growth of a transformed cell.

U

ultraviolet radiation Electromagnetic radiation with energy higher than that of visible light but less than that of X-rays.

unleaded gasoline Gasoline that does not contain the additive tetraethyllead.

unsaturated fat A fat whose molecules have carbon−carbon double bonds in their hydrocarbon chains.

unsaturated fatty acid A fatty acid possessing one or more double bonds between the carbons in the hydrocarbon tail.

uranium U; element 92 of the periodic table; uranium-235 is used as a nuclear fuel and explosive.

V

vaccine   A harmless variant or derivative of a pathogen that stimulates a host's immune system to mount defenses against the pathogen.

vapor   The gaseous state of a substance.

vasodilator   A chemical that causes blood vessels to dilate and lowers the blood pressure.

vegetable oil   Fat derived from a plant.

vinegar   5% solution of acetic acid in water.

visible light   That portion of the electromagnetic spectrum detected as various colors by the human eye, ranging in wavelength from about 400 nm (nanometers) to about 700 nm.

vision   The photochemical process by which humans and animals see.

vitamin   An organic molecule required in the diet in very small amounts; vitamins serve primarily as coenzymes or parts of coenzymes.

vitamin A   Retinol; deficiency causes night blindness; vitamin A is the precursor of retinal, the light-absorbing molecule in rhodopsin.

vitamin B   A complex set of molecules; deficiency causes a range of nervous disorders and anemia.

vitamin C   Ascorbic acid; deficiency causes scurvy.

vitamin D   Calciferol; deficiency causes rickets.

vitamin E   Tocopherol; deficiency causes a lack of hemoglobin in the blood.

W

wavelength   The distance between crests of waves, such as waves of the electromagnetic spectrum.

wax   A high-melting hydrocarbon.

weight   A measure of the gravitational force on a mass.

X

X-rays   Electromagnetic radiation with energy higher than that of ultraviolet light but less than that of γ-rays. The wavelengths of X-rays are about the same as the distances between atoms.

Y

yeast   A unicellular fungus that lives in liquid or moist habitats, primarily reproducing asexually by simple cell division or by budding of a parent cell.

Z

zinc   Zn; element 30 of the periodic table.

zinc oxide   ZnO; a mild base and a white pigment used in sunblocks.

Index

259

Index